Combat Radiology

Les R. Folio

Combat Radiology

Diagnostic Imaging of Blast and Ballistic Injuries

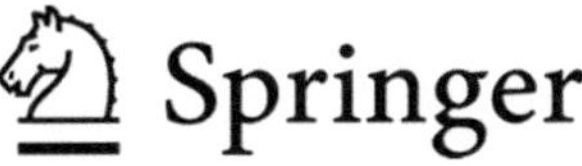 Springer

Les R. Folio, DO, MPH, FAOCR
Col (ret), USAF, MC, SFS
Associate Professor
Radiology and Radiological Sciences
Associate Professor
Military and Emergency Medicine
Uniformed Services
University of the Health Sciences
Bethesda, MD
USA

ISBN 978-1-4939-4047-9   ISBN 978-1-4419-5854-9 (eBook)
DOI 10.1007/978-1-4419-5854-9
Springer New York Heidelberg Dordrecht London

Springer is part of Springer Science+Business Media (www.springer.com)

To my wife, Jutta Frankfurter, and my son,
Lucas Skye Folio.

Foreword

I was certainly pleased when Dr. Les Folio invited me to write the foreword to his new textbook. We have been friends for many years and shared our understanding of biomechanics and imaging of high-energy trauma as well as our diagnostic approaches. We share a similar level of enthusiasm to maximize the diagnostic potential of imaging in severe trauma and to optimize conditions to facilitate faster and more accurate diagnoses, when time is the most critical commodity of care. We discovered many overlaps in our practice methods, but not surprising, many unique aspects to each.

Dr. Folio is a diplomat of the American Osteopathic Board of Radiology and American Osteopathic Board of Occupational and Preventive Medicine attaining Fellowship in both areas. He has earned master's degrees in Public Health, Clinical Radiology, and Aviation Sciences. He has served as an Air Force Radiologist and Flight Surgeon and recently completed 20 years in the Air Force; his final assignment was at Walter Reed Army Medical Center and Uniformed Services University (USU). He is an Associate Professor of Radiology and Radiological Sciences and Associate Professor of Military and Emergency Medicine at USU. He has completed tours of duty in Iraq and has contributed his knowledge in forensic radiology at Dover Air Force Base in Dover, Delaware, studying warfare. If these many significant accomplishments were not enough, he has also earned a black belt from World Taekwondo Federation while stationed in Korea and is a certified Master Scuba Diver and a lifetime member of National Ski Patrol. Relating his other major accomplishments would require another chapter in the book.

Clearly, Dr. Folio brings his diverse training and an inquisitive, creative mind to improving diagnostic imaging of the severely injured battlefield casualty. He uses his substantial knowledge of imaging, anatomy, and biomechanics to optimize the treatment of these patients and to constantly learn more to better understand high-energy force injury and possible methods to ameliorate their impact. In this process, he finds new questions that require further investigation. No one in America today has been better trained and experienced to write this text.

The reader of this text has a ringside seat to the unique imaging theater fashioned from the special medical demands of war. Dr. Folio shares many concepts that can be used in their entirety or adapted to the world of civilian trauma. Radiologists and other physicians, technologists, nurses, and ancillary medical support personnel caring for patients with penetrating and severe blunt force injury in their practices will benefit from reading this text.

Of course, the focus of this book is the imaging presentation of a variety of ballistic and blast injuries typical of battlefield wounding. An improved understanding of the medical effects and anatomic pathology created by ballistic missiles in all body regions is provided. The importance and methodology of establishing injury tracts through the body in deciding management are emphasized.

There are several chapters that discuss issues more generally applicable to major trauma on the home front. Many issues relevant to Emergency-Trauma Imaging are considered in this book. What "shortcuts" can be used to adequately image the major blunt force and penetrating trauma patient without sacrificing the accuracy of diagnosis? How are imaging protocols tailored to allow fast interpretation and transfer of vital information? How do we best integrate Radiology into the trauma team to assist in optimal triage and subsequent patient care? What are the major indications for advanced imaging applications such as volume rendering and CT angiography in a mass casualty setting? How best are technologists trained and supervised to perform rapid studies of optimal image quality? How are standardized reporting formats used to consistently provide reports containing all necessary information? What types of standard equipment modifications might be of value to more rapidly and efficiently image these patients?

Besides discussing the various technical issues in obtaining and interpreting battlefield images, Dr. Folio, who has a wealth of military medical experience, tells the reader a story of what it is like to serve as a military radiologist in this very demanding and stressful environment, but while also serving with a medical team at the height of collaboration and uniformity of purpose. I think you will enjoy and learn from his insights. The radiologist reader may acquire a whole new perspective on what a demanding workload really means. I expect that some of the ideas presented herein will find their way into many of the readers' practices. Enjoy!

Stuart E. Mirvis, MD
Professor of Radiology
University of Maryland School of Medicine

Preface

When I was invited by Springer to write this book on my experiences as a radiologist in Iraq, I immediately agreed (after consulting with my wife Jutta, of course) as it seemed the perfect "summer project" to fill the gap between retirement from the Air Force and starting my new career at the National Institutes of Health (NIH). The publisher found many of my publications on combat imaging, and since I had chaired several national and international conferences on trauma imaging, I was ready to put this book together in a short period of time. Our goal was to get the information out there for deploying radiologists to use and prepare for combat radiology. At the same time, I wanted to keep the book general enough to be a reference for any hospital with an emergency department or trauma unit since explosions, disasters, and mass casualties can happen at any time. Since ballistic injuries are often the unintended consequences anywhere man and guns collide, this book should be generalizable to most radiologists, emergency department physicians, trauma unit nurses/medics, and trauma surgeons worldwide.

Once I started writing, this book evolved differently than what I had originally envisioned. After discussions with many of my colleagues and friends, however, it seemed the resulting format is better than a systems-based approach that I had first planned. Those reading my initial drafts suggested that I capture the essence of the environment from the beginning and do not use a head-to-toe approach.

To set the stage, I included a background on what it is like for a radiologist to be in the military and have to deploy into harm's way at a moment's notice, what it is like to carry a weapon at all times, and what it is like to wear body armor and a helmet while consulting trauma surgeons on images, all while being attacked.

Following a description of combat scenes, to the layout of our combat hospital, I then decided to describe basic blast and ballistic properties both outside and inside the body. For example, I felt that showing photos I had taken during medical effects of blast in field tests in South Africa would show how extensive blast damage can be, even when made with basic materials. After discussing the types of explosives and the types of blast injuries, I then show some example images of patients exposed to different types of blast.

A combat-unique chapter further sets the scene of battlefield radiology and prepares one for the innovation and creativity necessary to help as many casualties as possible, when resources are strained. Several new medical ideas, concepts, and patented inventions have emerged from prior conflicts. Recent wars have achieved record-breaking lifesaving statistics. For example, our combat hospital had a 98% survival rate during our deployment in 2007, the highest recorded to that point. Many revolutionary technologies and processes contributed to these unprecedented proportions. I will touch on new tourniquets and their application: Air Evacuation, FAST and E-FAST, MDCT with 3D and MPR processing to include trajectory analysis, and APS (Anatomic Positioning System, like an anatomic GPS). Many of these concepts are still evolving, while others are patent-pending inventions in imaging advances, awaiting field implementation.

I believe that imaging is contributing significantly to determining salvageability of life, limb, and eyesight. Sharing our experiences with war casualties, with the most advanced imaging capabilities, will allow further progress in helping determine morbidity and mortality over time from an epidemiological perspective. Standard reporting schemes on penetrating trauma should help compare radiologic data mining with clinical correlation over the years in a more quantitative fashion. I will discuss my experiences, research, and theories on standardized and quantitative reporting along with advances that will allow these to be automated in the near future. This will make radiologists more efficient while providing more detailed imaging finding descriptions in a standard fashion.

Les R. Folio, DO, MPH, FAOCR
Col (ret), USAF, MC, SFS

Acknowledgments

I would like to acknowledge Sofia Echelmeyer for her excellent artwork in several of the chapters. I thank the medical staff of the 332nd Medical Group for allowing me to serve them as a radiologist. Working with and under the Tuskegee Airman Wing in Iraq is the most rewarding experience a military doctor can have in my opinion. Additionally, I would like to thank Genevieve Jacobs for her exceptional editorial services. I further acknowledge the following people for their help with various chapters throughout this book: Dr. Rolf Bunger, Tatjana Fischer, Lt Chris Backus, Gerd Frankfurter, Bill Knepshield, Michael Frew, MD, David Cruea, Israel Felix, RT, David Stancil, Dr. Andy Dwyer, Anna Grefe, and Dominik Usling.

Contents

Chapter 1
The Combat Environment: Preparation for Deployment

Keywords Deployment · Center for the Sustainment of Trauma and Readiness Skills (CSTARS) · Echelons of care · Area of operations (AOR) · Combat support hospital · Air Force theater hospital

1.1 Introduction

The environment of a deployed combat hospital brings many challenges such as artillery fire, heat, sand, dust, cold, and frequent power outages. This chapter will provide an overview of deployment preparation and battlefield challenges the military radiologist needs to know. In addition, the concepts and cases presented here should provide baseline knowledge for mass casualty/disaster preparation for any radiologist where there is an emergency room.

Trauma imaging in the combat environment parallels civilian radiology from a procedural and pathologic perspective. There are some very unique aspects of diagnostic imaging in the deployed military setting, however, including desert conditions such as heat, sand, and dust. Conditions can also include cold, mountainous, or tropical environments. In addition, patient care continues with daily power outages, combat operations, explosions, ducking in bunkers from incoming artillery fire and indirect insurgent fire, often working with cumbersome body armor. It is not unusual during continual patient care that technologists have to check for unexploded ordinance outside the department after being fired upon (daily for our tour of duty). The overarching principles of care in theater are greatly influenced by a combat environment that is very resource-limited. This is a fact that enters into every diagnostic consideration and treatment decision.

In addition to trauma and emergency care image findings seen in the US, combat unique images will be presented with representative cases in areas such as blast and high velocity missile injury as well as heroic diagnostics and therapeutics typically only seen on the battlefield. This may serve as a reference in disaster preparedness for US institutions and teaching programs in addition to university hospitals and medical centers. The information in this chapter should be generalizable to civilian

L. Folio (ed.), *Combat Radiology: Diagnostic Imaging of Blast and Ballistic Injuries*,
DOI 10.1007/978-1-4419-5854-9_1, © Springer Science+Business Media, LLC 2010

hospitals, not just trauma centers, but also the most remote [1] community hospital in America that may see the most severe trauma at any time.

Hopefully when reading this book, however, one will appreciate how we solved the problem and made up for limitations and challenges that are not traditionally encountered and would not even be considered in civilian settings, except in extreme conditions. For example, skipping the portable CXR in the ED and obtaining it on the CT scout; screening through the entire chest/abdomen/pelvis on one universal wide window in seconds to provide an overview of life threatening injuries; or compressing Gigabytes of data into megabytes (100:1 compression) and emailing mp4 videos to provide another facility a prior exam to be available. Another seemingly bold effort to answer the longitudinal medical record challenge being investigated is a personal health vault solution with uploadable compressed CT movie files online. Although the military pioneered teleradiology [2, 3] and electronic health records, increasing security requirements have severely hampered the possibility of compatible medical records and paper, e-mail, and CDs of images still being used.

1.2 Preparation for Deployment

Radiologists in the military, whether active or reservist, know that deployment is a real possibility and are often already prepared from a physical and mental perspective. Depending on where a radiologist is stationed, there are variable times and chances of being deployed. Once a radiologist is in the window of potential deployment, there are military specific requirements that need to be met. These include making sure annual immunizations are current (to include area specific immunization), annual (or bi-annual) physical fitness tests are passed, annual physical examination is completed, pistol (M9 and/or M14/M16) training is current, and that chemical, biological, and radiological warfare training is updated often prior to notification of a deployment.

1.3 Personal Effects

In addition to training for preparation for combat conditions and gathering of military specific equipment, there are personal items to strategically pack to prepare oneself for 4–6 (potentially 15) months of living in combat conditions. Figure 1.1 shows the bags I packed on my first deployment to Iraq to include military gear, personal items, a 72 h pack (the green backpack on top), and a carry-on backpack with reading material and laptop. Many experienced deployers will mark their luggage with shiny or fluorescent markers to help pick out their luggage in overseas staging airports. This helps find luggage since there are no baggage handlers; you have to find your own bags among everyone else, usually at night, outside.

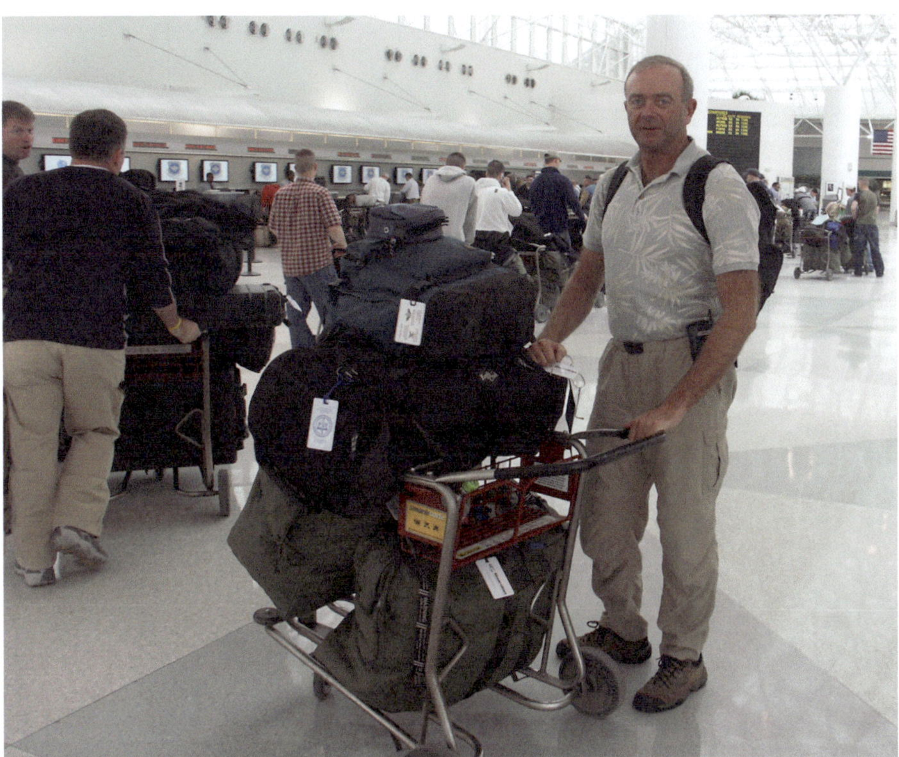

Fig. 1.1 This photo was taken of me just prior to my first deployment to Iraq back in 2005. Note the two military *green bags* on the bottom; they were for chemical gear, body armor, helmet, etc. My weapon was already checked in at this point

See Fig. 1.2 of myself arriving in Balad, Iraq in a C17 after almost a week of travel on my second deployment to Iraq.

It takes weeks to receive care packages from home if something is overlooked, however, there are limited supplies sold in military stores, even in combat zones (especially where radiologists typically deploy). Military specific items necessary include helmet, body armor, weapon (M-9 or Beretta), uniforms, boots, chemical warfare gear (suit, gas mask, filters, chemical agent antidotes), self aide medical kits, etc. Mostly, everything is issued (free) to active duty and civilian contractors; however, many spend hundreds or thousands of dollars on equipment above what is issued.

Many experienced deployed military personnel use sweater/shoe organizers to maximize the small space; one must pack all their gear to have ready at a moments notice. Since there are often delays and layovers in traveling, it is imperative to have a 72 h bag prepared to live out of without digging into the four or five bags you may be traveling with. For example, we got delayed due to massive deployments and aircraft breakdown for about 100 h; so our 72 h kits (two changes of civilian clothes/shoes, shower kit) overextended themselves.

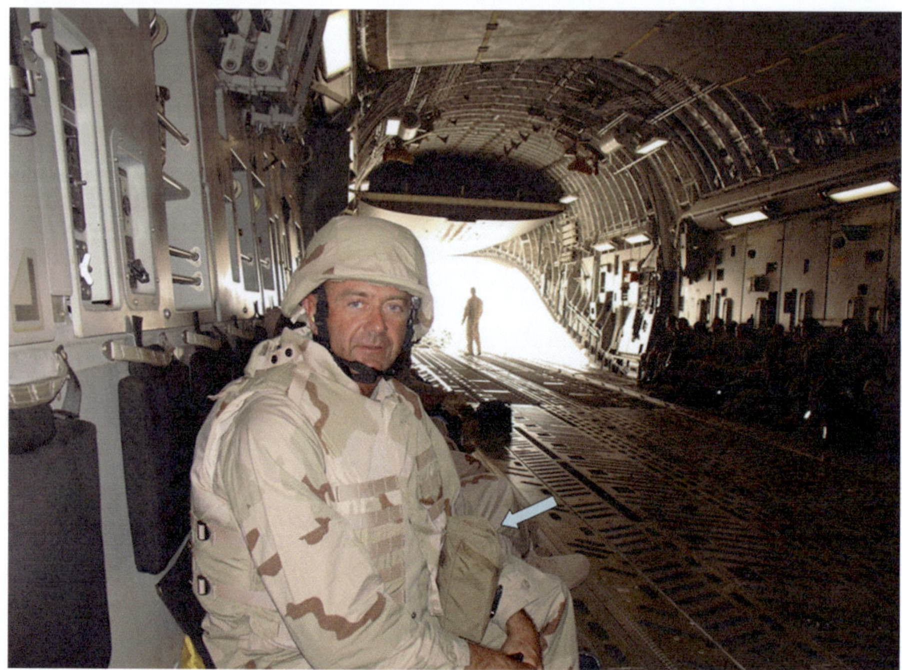

Fig. 1.2 Note the body armor and self-aide medical kit (*arrow*) everyone deploys with. We also carry our weapons, chemical warfare gear/gas mask, antidotes, and additional equipment.

Since I am also a flight surgeon and most often deploy in that capacity, I bring additional items most radiologists would not need. However, I think it is useful to have access to a short medication list that has helped me as a flight surgeon and a radiologist on deployments where I was the only doctor for several hundred deploying personnel. One must keep in mind that one travels with different groups of deployers; many times none are medical and you may be the only medical trained professional with hundreds of people that may turn to you for medical advice of all kinds. See the following reference for a list of medications that have served me well to have on hand for about eight deployments to include Bolivia, Saudi Arabia, Turkey, and the South Pole [4].

1.4 Military Training for Deployment

The moment a radiologist is officially tasked with an upcoming deployment, further training and preparation must be completed. Traditionally, most training and preparation at this point is military-specific and not necessarily related to the everyday job. As the time to depart gets closer, online and other training include hostile environment preparation, equipment gathering, instructions on how to

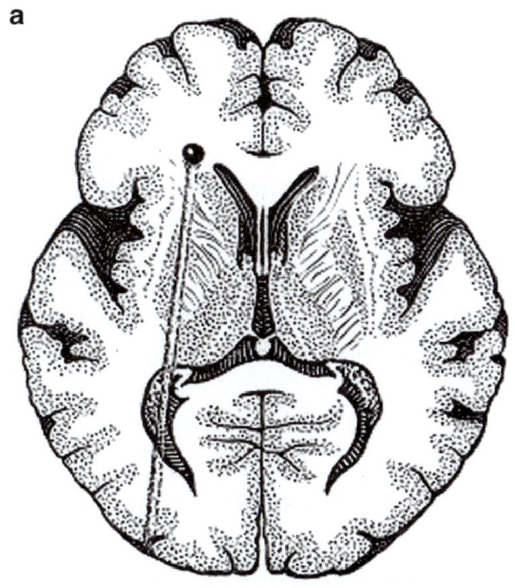

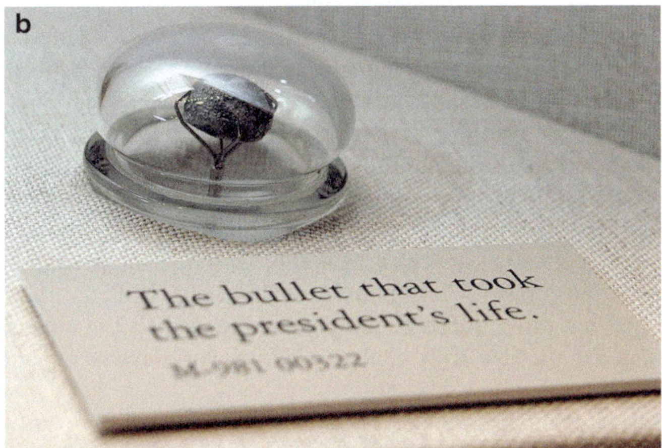

Fig. 1.2 (continued) (**a**) Artist drawing of an axial slice (not dissimilar to a modern-day CT slice) is housed in the National Museum of Health and Medicine, Armed Forces Institute of Pathology, Washington, D.C. (founded, ironically, by President Lincoln on May 12, 1862). Donated graciously with permission to reprint by the National Museum of Health and Medicine, Armed Forces Institute of Pathology. (**b**) This photo is of the bullet that killed President Lincoln on April 15, 1865. It was removed at autopsy in the White House by Army Medical Museum surgeons Lt. Col. Joseph Woodward and Major Edward Curtis and is still. This is a photo of the display at the National Museum of Health and Medicine, Armed Forces Institute of Pathology, Washington, D. C. Donated graciously with permission to reprint by the National Museum of Health and Medicine, Armed Forces Institute of Pathology

prepare military paperwork, personal items such as wills and paying bills while away, etc. Time for specific training for the work a radiologist does in combat is typically overlooked and pushed to the side as other tasks become more apparent and overwhelm the deploying member. Training for an Air Force radiologist for example, occurs once they arrive in the theater of operations. At that point, it is too late to brush up on any skills or learn the specifics of penetrating trauma, workflow in a combat hospital, understand military specific terminology, among others.

All military members, to include all doctors, are provided basic survival courses in the beginning of their career. There are additional optional environmental survival courses in the military (winter, arctic, water, mountain, jungle, etc.), however, these are generally reserved for more operational military positions (pilots, flight surgeons, civil engineers, infantry, etc.).

1.5 Trauma and Critical Care Imagining Training

At the larger military hospitals where several radiologists have deployed experience, those preparing for deployment have an opportunity to obtain informal preparation. Radiologists stationed in smaller medical facilities (such as superclinics) do not have those advantages and often seek other means of honing trauma skills or getting refreshed before deploying. Taking vacation time is often necessary to visit trauma level 1 facilities to experience the flow, pace, and techniques. Some will become familiar on the equipment they will be working on by going to hospitals that have similar equipment. For example, not every hospital performs MultiPlanar Reformation (MPR), Maximum Intensity Projections (MIP), or 3D volumetric reconstructions on a regular basis. These are performed on a daily basis in combat hospitals as this book will highlight. Military radiologists are generally aware that using different equipment when starting in new hospitals can be challenging. Familiarity with vendor specific workflow is imperative before fluency is gained.

Other informal training includes exposure in busy civilian or military trauma centers for days to weeks. Unfortunately, this is often on the radiologists' own time since there is no formal mechanism in place to allow for radiologists' absence from their current jobs to visit other hospitals. While stationed at USU, I overhauled an existing readiness skills verification website for minimal training requirements for deploying radiologists [5]. I developed a curriculum, included my After Action Report (AAR) based on experiences in Iraq, to include equipment used and trauma protocols. I also included a quiz with images and multiple casualty scenarios. We also developed an imaging trauma simulator using PowerPoint, including cases to accompany manikin simulators at our annual Bushmaster exercise, first used in 2008. As students are challenged with simulators that stop breathing, pulse, and interact with ACLS protocols, unknown X-rays and CT images are presented to simulate CXR, pelvis, CT to take scenarios to the next level.

1.6   Air Force Radiologist Training

Formal trauma training for radiologists is under development to include a draft curriculum and course at R Adams Cowley Shock Trauma Center in Baltimore. This could fall under the existing deploying course structure called CSTARS. This stands for Center for the Sustainment of Trauma and Readiness Skills and is for deploying physicians, nurses, and medics, however, has not traditionally included radiologists. This has recently changed and a CSTARS-R (CSTARS-Radiologists) trial course has begun at Baltimore Shock Trauma. This 3 week course will be taught by trauma surgeons and radiologists to help prepare radiologists for deployment. I spent 4 years pushing for a course for deploying radiologists, and it finally became a reality by the time I retired from the Air Force in 2009.

One radiology technique that pushed me to advocate a course such as the CSTARS-R program was the identification of ballistic wound paths using our new MDCT. The images that we obtained allowed us to diagnose and treat hundreds of penetrating ballistic injuries. I was afraid that without a course to teach inbound radiologists how to assess ballistic injuries, many casualties would go improperly treated. As battlefield imaging became more advanced, deployed military radiologists were becoming increasingly convinced that ballistic injuries were more detectable than ever before. My second deployment to Iraq in 2007 was timely in that the scanners used were to be among the first multi-slice CTs on the battlefield. Weeks after the first MDCTs were on the front lines; it seemed that radiologists were desperately trying to pass on the valuable knowledge regarding wounds paths. This significantly aided our trauma surgeons when deciding who to triage to the operating room. We used the wound path to identify injuries that may have gone unrecognized otherwise. We know that when it comes to penetrating head trauma, real estate is everything (location, location, location). In addition, it is known that trajectory determination helps in critical organ identification in the abdomen [6, 7]. For example, one of the major criteria for determining a diaphragm injury was highlighted by Sliker in 2006. Sliker determined that the trajectory/ path of a missile or knife raises suspicion of a diaphragm injury [8,9].

Let us take trajectory analysis a step further, rather than forward in time, back to 1865, the assassination of President Lincoln. After being shot in the back of the head at Ford's theater, he was tended to by several physicians and surgeons that knew his condition was grave (hours to live). See Fig. 1.2a for the trajectory best mapped out by the scientific medical knowledge at the time. Had President Lincoln been rushed to the nearest trauma facility and undergone a CT, based on my experience, he would not have survived despite medical advances. There has been some vector analysis in neurotrauma that supports injury to the area in this drawing that indicates this is a fatal injury by Kim et al. [10]. They had termed the terminus of this ballistic as the "zona fatalis" in that in their study, all injuries to this area were fatal. See Fig. 1.2b for the bullet that ended the President's life. The AFIP, originally called the Army Medical Museum, was founded by President Abraham Lincoln on its original mission to collect pathological specimens and case histories of Civil War soldiers to facilitate research to improve wartime medicine.

In Chap. 5, I will highlight recent research on wound path identification and trajectory analysis; to the point where radiologists can help scene investigators in identifying the direction a sniper shot from (for example), or the location and strength of a bomb blast based on the fragment patterns in the body from CT imaging.

1.7 Radiology Equipment Challenges

There are challenges in combat environments that make running complicated radiology equipment 24–7 difficult. Weather and climate conditions make the logistics and maintenance of CT (for example) a constant challenge. Overseas power sources are often 50 cycles instead of 60 cycles, and are not often 220 V. Local outlets are not standard US; however, facilities are built similar to US, thanks to military engineers and logistics personnel. At the time of this writing, there is no role for MRI in combat conditions. With high turnover rates of personnel, number of casualties with metallic fragments in unpredictable locations, a compromise of ferromagnetic hygiene would be inevitable. In addition, the support is not available to maintain MRI in combat conditions.

See Fig. 1.3 to highlight the dusty environment of the tent facility. This was the radiologist reading room before moving to the new hardened facility in 2007. There

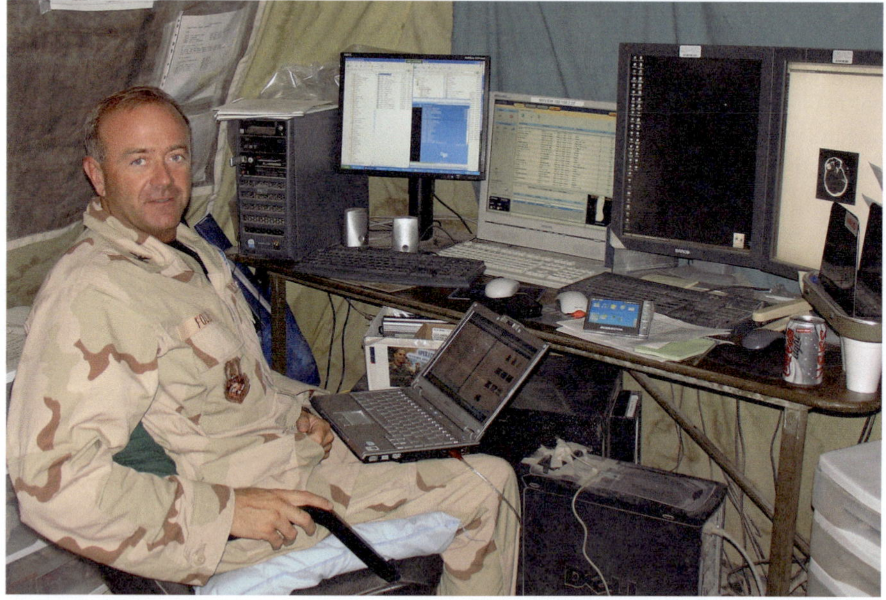

Fig. 1.3 Radiologist reading room in the tent facility. Note the sand/dust over much of the equipment

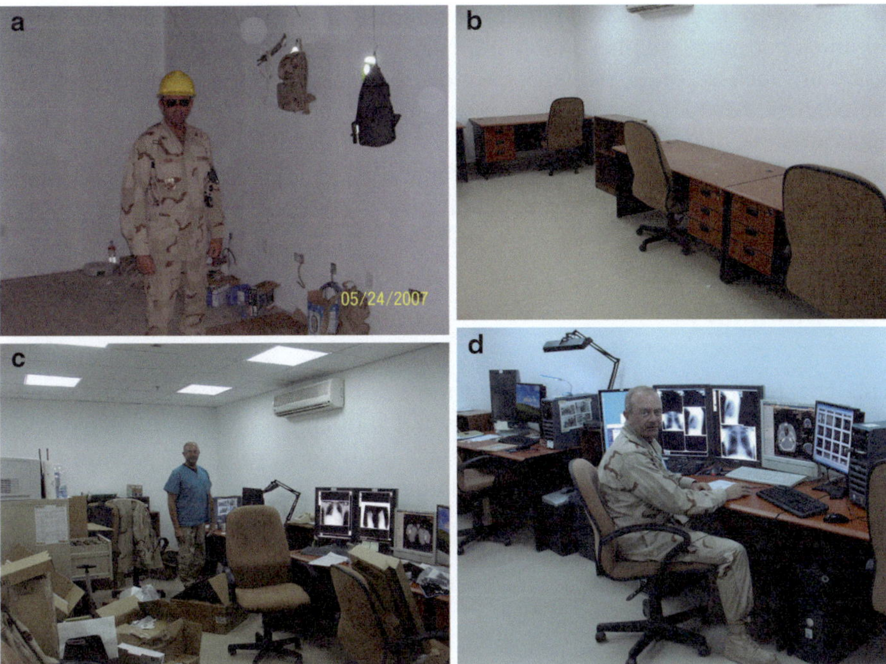

Fig. 1.4 (**a–d**) Putting together the new reading room while building the new facility

were times during sand storms that the entire reading room was filled with dust and one had to wear goggles to see just a few feet. This was remedied after moving to the new facility; see Fig. 1.4a–d for the building of the new reading room. As Chief of Radiology, I made sure there was radiologist input in the location and design of the reading room and efficient flow of patients through the radiology department.

1.8   Redeployment, Preparation to Return Home

Lastly, one needs to consider how to prepare to redeploy, or return home. This may seem trivial compared to preparing to deploy in the first place, however, there are many items to consider. There are five stages of military deployment: predeployment, deployment, sustainment, redeployment, and postdeployment. One must be proactive in preparing their own flight home by providing any specifics about their orders and base that deployed them. Allowing work to overwhelm, you can precipitate an item being overlooked, causing delay in flights back home (for example). There are home preparations that need to be arranged and family back home is not used to having the military member around [11].

One common problem shared by many returning military personnel is driving or being a passenger in a car. Deployed military are limited to small bases with little driving experience. Even when driving on a small deployed base, speeds are below 30 miles per hour. Another problem medical providers have is how trivial many issues are such as forms, red tape, even cases seemingly exciting to many civilian radiologists. Tolerance to seemingly mundane tasks is significantly lowered. Lastly, once out of the desert, colors seem vivid and unreal since one is used to desert sand, drab uniforms, and military setting. The intensity of the colors almost seems like a visual overload; with difficulty explaining how much color we have in the US. I believe some of us take what we have in America for granted.

1.9 Summary

This chapter has hopefully introduced the combat hospital setting, painting the picture of the radiologists' life in this new and unusual world. Before a deployment to a combat zone, there are basic challenges of what to pack and prepare for, in addition to all the military clothing and equipment. The challenges of preparing mentally and physically for deployment were discussed. This chapter should set the scene for upcoming chapters to provide a feel for limitations and challenges and how they were dealt with and expansion of creativity necessary to work in such hostile and austere environments.

References

1. Folio LR, Hanson E, Chao S. Generalizability of US air force studies: 1990 and 2000 demographic distribution comparison of US active duty air force personnel and the US general population. Mil Med 2002 Nov;167(11):911–9.
2. Folio L, Stokes R, Frankfurter J. From film to filmless: military experience with teleradiology in Korea. Appl Radiol, July 95. 36–39.
3. Cade LD, Leckie RG, Goeringer F. MDIS (Medical Diagnostic Imaging Support): the new standard in filmless imaging. Adm Radiol 1993 Nov;12(11):59–61.
4. Deploying flight surgeon medication list. http://rad.usuhs.mil/rad/handouts/folio/SME_-Drug_List_Sept2004.xls Accessed August 15, 2009.
5. Readiness skills verification webpage; uniformed services university. http://rad.usuhs.mil/project44R3/index.html Accessed August 12, 2009.
6. Shanmuganathan K, Mirvis SE, Chiu WC, et al. Penetrating torso trauma: triple-contrast helical CT in peritoneal violation and organ injury – a prospective study in 220 patients. Radiology 2004;231(3):775–84.
7. Larici AR, Gotway MB, Litt HI, et al. Helical CT with sagittal and coronal reconstructions: accuracy for detection of diaphragmatic injury. AJR Am J Roentgenol 2002;179:451–7.
8. Sliker CW. Imaging of diaphragm injuries. Radiol Clin North Am 2006;44(2):199–211, vii.
9. Steenburg SD, Sliker CW, Shanmuganathan K, Siegel EL. Imaging evaluation of penetrating neck injuries. Radiograph 2010 Jul-Aug;30(4):869-86.
10. Kim KA, Wang MY, McNatt SA, Pinsky G, Liu CY, Giannotta SL, Apuzzo ML. Vector analysis correlating bullet trajectory to outcome after civilian through-and-through gunshot wound to the head: using imaging cues to predict fatal outcome. Neurosurgery 2005 Oct;57 (4):737–47; discussion 737–47.
11. Fitzsimons VM, Krause-Parello CA. Military children: when parents are deployed overseas. J Sch Nurs 2009 Feb;25(1):40-7.

Chapter 2
Echelons of Combat Casualty Care and Associated Imaging Resources

Keywords Logistics · Echelons · Levels of combat casualty care · Air Force Theater Hospital · Combat Support Hospital · Biomedical Equipment Technicians · Area of operations · Composite Health Care System · Joint Patient Tracking System

2.1 Introduction

This chapter provides an overview of the various levels and capabilities of hospitals in deployed military bases in combat zones. This includes the equipment and staffing resources, capabilities, and roles in the flow of combat casualty care. The major role of radiologists in the combat setting is at Level 3 facilities. The equipment at our Level 3 facility in Balad, Iraq, will serve as an example of resources available at most other Level 3 facilities in Iraq and Afghanistan.

2.2 Echelons of Care

There are five echelons of care from the front lines through Germany and back to CONUS (Continental US). There is some variation based on experiences at each of the bases, and additional equipment that may be acquired after initial laydown.

The first echelon is referred to as self-aide buddy care (taking care of oneself, or another) on the battlefield. All nonmedical and medical military are taught techniques for saving themselves or others with tourniquets, large bandages for massive lacerations, BLS, etc.

The second echelon (Level 2) is a small hospital with basic surgical and imaging capability, usually without a radiologist. This has varied a bit, for example, in Mosul, Iraq, where there has been a radiologist in the past, and a CT (usually, there is a radiologist where there is CT, but not always). There is basic plain radiography and ultrasound, to sometimes include C-arm and portable units.

L. Folio (ed.), *Combat Radiology: Diagnostic Imaging of Blast and Ballistic Injuries*, DOI 10.1007/978-1-4419-5854-9_2, © Springer Science+Business Media, LLC 2010

The Level 3 facilities have a radiologist (up to three), CT (at least one), and basic plain radiography, ultrasound, trauma surgery, ICU, and wards. Some Level 3 facilities (such as ours) have subspecialists.

Level 4 facilities are major overseas hospitals that include Landstuhl Army Medical Center in Germany, (see Fig. 2.1) and Tripler Army Hospital in Hawaii. These hospitals are well-equipped major medical centers that would rival many US trauma centers and university hospitals.

The final Level 5 hospitals are major receiving hospitals in the US and include Walter Reed Army Medical Center in Washington, DC (see Fig. 2.2), Brook Army Hospital and Wilford Hall Medical Center in San Antonio, TX, and David Grant Medical Center in California.

Much of the content of this book will include cases from a Level 3 Air Force Theater Hospital (AFTH) in Balad, Iraq, approximately 60 miles north of Baghdad. (see Fig. 2.3) for an example of a Level 3 tent facility in Iraq. The flow of trauma in combat hospitals is similar to trauma centers in the United States, except with much more volume and percentage of major trauma. The helipad in Balad is capable of receiving four helicopters at one time, each with up to six patients. The casualties are transported to the Emergency Department and triaged (sometimes just outside the ED) for CT and OR. (see Fig. 2.4a) showing the Emergency Department in the tent facility in Balad, Iraq. A section of the floor (known as "Bay 2") of this well-known ED has been transported to the National Museum of Health and Medicine of the Armed Forces Institute of Pathology (NMHM, Fig. 2.4b) [1]. Bay 2 saw the most serious of injuries since it was in closest proximity to the operating rooms. There was a Bay 1, however, the portable X-ray unit took that space over time.

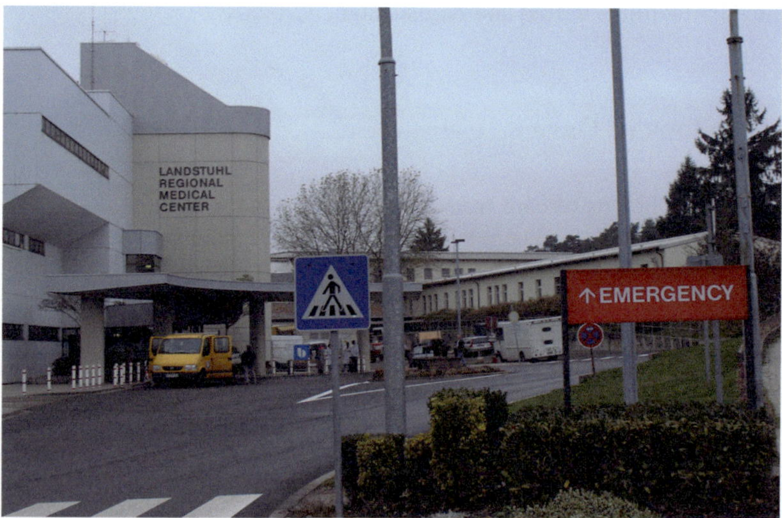

Fig. 2.1 The emergency room entrance and receiving point for combat casualties air-evacuated for more definitive care. Photo by Dr. Les Folio

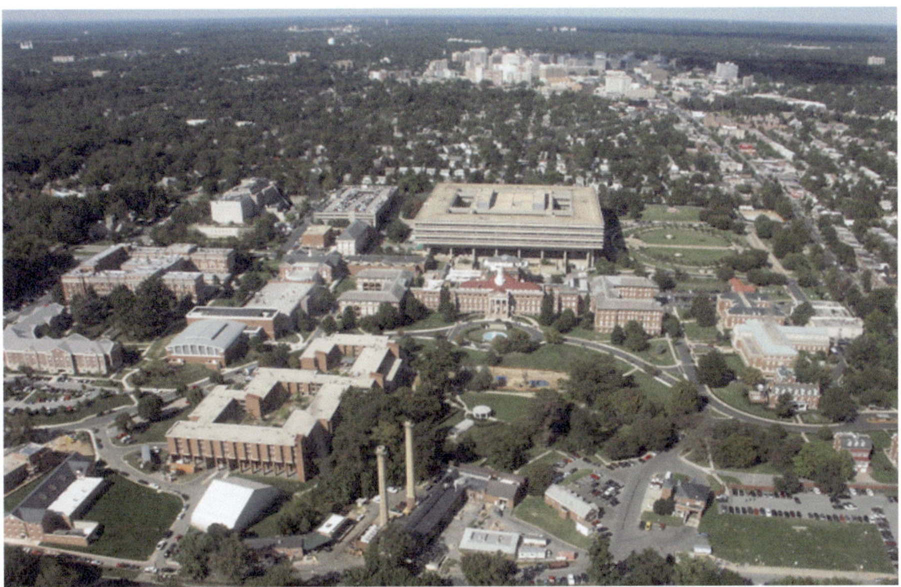

Fig. 2.2 Walter Reed Army Medical Center, a major Level 5 facility in the US. Photo by Dr. Les Folio

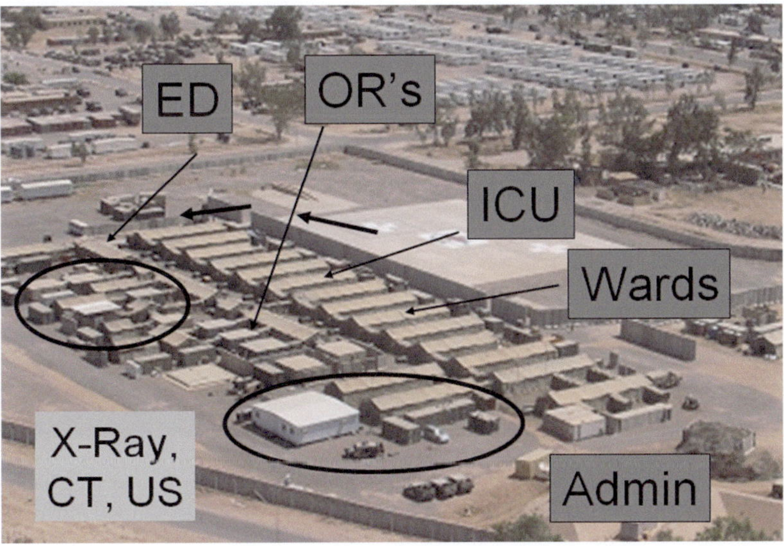

Fig. 2.3 This photo shows the tent configuration where the majority of cases presented in this book were treated. This was located in Balad, Iraq and housed a Level 3 Air Force Theater Hospital. Casualties arrive on the large helipad, then quickly moved to the ED by NATO litters (*arrows*), then to CT/OR, then ICU and wards before being evacuated to Germany

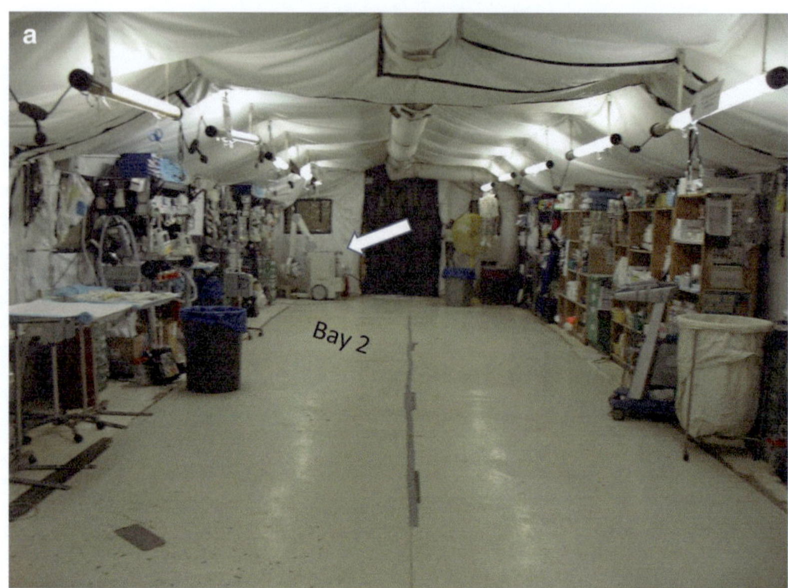

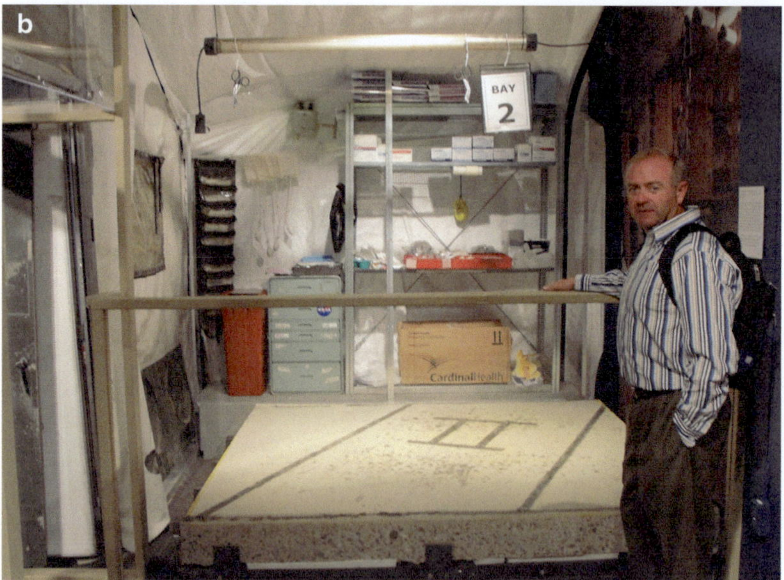

Fig. 2.4 (**a**) This emergency department had seen thousands of severely wounded casualties from 2004 to 2007. (**b**) Photo of Bay 2 on display at the National Museum of Health and Medicine of the Armed Forces Institute of Pathology in Washington, DC

2.3 Imaging Resources at a Level 3 Facility

Most of the cases reviewed in this book are from the tent facility before moving to the hardened facility late in our rotation. The capabilities were basically the same, with some improvements in equipment and software after the move. For more information about the move to the new facility, see my description in Military Medical Technology of challenges we faced of moving a radiology department while under hostile fire [2]. We moved the hospital while not closing our doors to major combat trauma.

2.3.1 Radiology Staffing, Hours

Our deployed radiology department had eight registered radiologic technologists (six AF, two Army) and three radiologists. For a photo of our department and more information, see a brief overview of our technologists work and experience in the RT journal [3]. It should be kept in mind that there is no requirement to deploy CT technologists (not that I agree to that tradition). Most techs are not experienced with CT and get their training in that 3-day turnover period previously mentioned.

I believe several technologists be specifically trained on CT, and all deploying techs have some basic CT experience. One technologist should be trained in ultrasound, and three in general radiology. We trained our general technologists to perform CT and had no problem in getting all techs up to speed on performing studies. Even the ultrasound technologist did CT for more than half of each day. The predominant need is for CT training, see Figs. 2.5 and 2.6 for an example of our CT in an isoshelter. Our ability to tailor studies was limited, however, by the lack of CT training. We were fortunate to have a trained ultrasound technologist, with the result that ultrasound use increased by 65%, supporting the benefit of having this skill set in theater.

We performed around 15,000 radiology exams in 4 months. The medical group hospital was called the 332nd Expeditionary Medical Group, and the radiology department was referred to as the Radiology Flight. We provided medical imaging for the AFTH, two Army clinics at Camp Anaconda, and several theater clinics. We also provided imaging services to outlying forward operating bases (FOB). We imaged most patients coming through our facility staging from other bases in preparation for evacuation to LRMC.

Radiologists worked in 8 h shifts (7a–3p, 3p–11p, and 11p–7a). We were fortunate to have three radiologists, as initial rotations had only two and were often overwhelmed and tired. We worked 7 days a week, rotating shifts twice during the cycle so that each radiologist worked each shift for about 6 weeks. We worked the first 80 days straight without a day off. This got a little old and we decided to double up on weekends to allow ourselves 2 days off a month. This schedule was manageable, with one difficulty being accessibility of the flight commander for meetings when working in the night shifts. We often overlapped

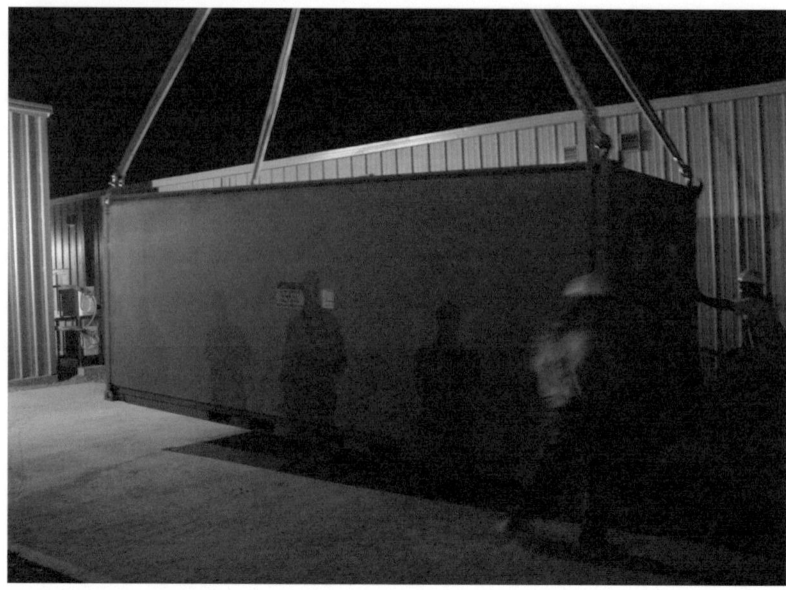

Fig. 2.5 Isoshelter containing a CT being carefully lowered to a concrete slab by a crane during the move to the new hardened facility. These isoshelters can provide operating room environments, large equipment such as CT or plain radiography rooms, and clean laboratories. Photo by Dr. Les Folio

schedules (i.e., night radiologist stayed for clinical radiology rounds, day radiologist left at 5 p.m., alloing two radiologists on duty for an hour) and stayed late when needed. The flight commander often worked longer hours due to administrative responsibilities such as daily meetings.

Given the volume and distribution of studies, each radiologist should be board-certified and have a current skill set in general body and trauma imaging as well as ultrasound scanning experience. Basic interventional radiology skills are useful but not essential as there were deployed vascular surgeons and neurosurgeons. There are a variety of radiology subspecialists that deploy, allowing expertise to spread for a well-rounded department. We were fortunate to have several continuous deployments with neuroradiologists/neurointerventional radiologists to allow for a continual supply and expertise in interventional techniques and equipment.

2.3.2 Radiology Equipment

We had two 16 Slice MD CTs, one diagnostic X-ray unit, two working portables, and one main US unit. Our CTs were two new (not a year old yet) 16-slice Philips Brilliance CT scanners. These clearly demonstrated their usefulness with their speed and detail. We used the prior rotations' detailed update of the imaging protocols in a CT protocol binder. We reviewed this, added a few programs, but the simplicity of

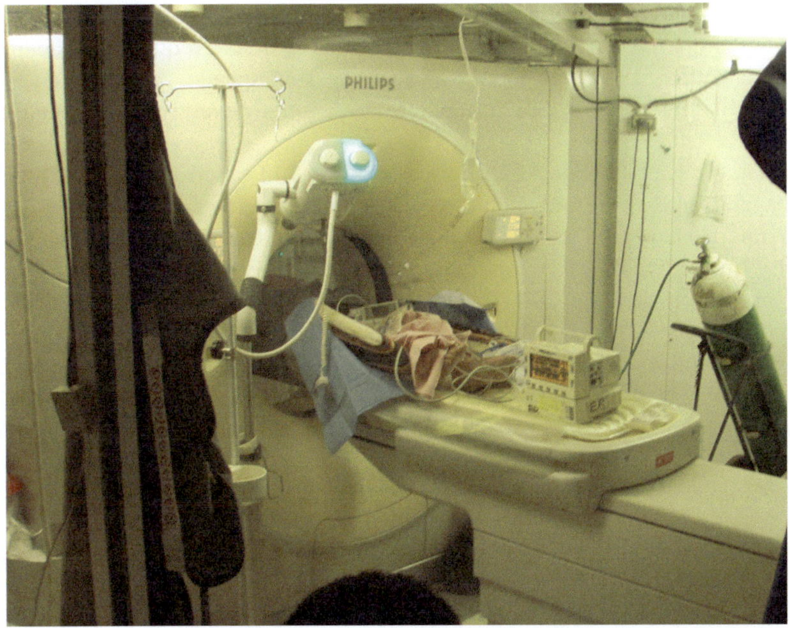

Fig. 2.6 One of our two MD CTs in an isoshelter. Note the portable life support equipment routinely placed at the foot of the patient. Many of our CT patients were on the border of hemodynamic stability. Photo by Dr. Les Folio

the protocols allowed for ease of use. The mechanics of each protocol were programmed into each scanner. Two Phillips Brilliance workstations were in use (one in the radiology department, and the other in the ED). A small satellite radiology reading area was created outside the ED for faster image reading during trauma codes. These workstations enabled radiologists to quickly review the CT images, even while the exam was still being acquired. The 3D volume rendering and additional tools were especially helpful and will be discussed in a dedicated chapter.

Previous radiologists that deployed recommended obtaining one backup CT tube for emergency replacement. Biomed tech familiarity with the Philips scanners and the vendor technical support team is essential. We were lucky to have experienced Biomedical Equipment Technicians (BMETS) that were always available and provided a 95% uptime. We continued to update and automate CT protocols, especially focusing on automatic image transmission since this was a constant challenge and moving target.

2.3.2.1 Orex Computed Radiography Readers

We started the rotation with two functioning Orex ACL4 Computed Radiography (CR) readers. Both units had new rollers installed during this cycle, which has greatly enhanced their reliability, but we learned to expect rapid degradation and were prepared to refurbish and repair these units frequently. The readers became a bottleneck due to their slower processing speeds. At times, one of the readers will malfunction, but fortunately both units never malfunctioned at the same time.

Two new faster OREX ACL6 processors were installed directly into the new facility, and one of the old scanners was maintained for continued use. The old reader has been placed alongside one of the new readers for use during mass-casualty operations or other rapid tempo periods. The second ACL6 processor is being placed outside the OR. The OREX brand is familiar to the BMET repair personnel.

High-resolution monitors were connected to the processing units for better initial interpretations of images. This significantly speeds up initial interpretations and provides the trauma surgeons an opportunity to review images quickly as per ATLS guidelines.

2.3.2.2 Portable/Fixed X-Ray Units

We arrived having three functional portable units and one backup portable unit. We would lend units out to local clinics when able, and tried keeping a few extras handy just in case. At no time were all portables down as this would have been cata-strophic. I believe a digital portable unit that instantly shows images on the unit's LCD screen upon exposure would be useful in increasing image availability during times when the network is overwhelmed. Such a unit was considered, however, these were not ready for prime time during our rotation. I would also recommend considering a StatScan (by Lodox) based on what I have seen at Baltimore Shock Trauma and visiting other hospitals with this expedient equipment [4, 5].

2.3.2.3 Ultrasound

We had one Sonosite MicroMaxx and one Sonosite Titan ultrasound unit. All units can be connected to the MedWeb for image archive and transmission. In addition, the Emergency Department has a SonoSite Titan, which they use for FAST scans. There were other US units owned by ED and ICU.

2.3.2.4 MedWeb and MedWeb Reading Stations

We used a PACS system vendor named MedWeb (San Francisco, CA). This system is used by the US Army and has electronic connections with some of the US Army Combat Support Hospitals (CSHs). We added a link to Mosul during our cycle. This system works well, but the electronic links to other CSHs are often nonfunctional due to network bandwidth problems and firewall blocking. Usually this means the outside study lists can be viewed, but studies cannot be pulled in. To get a specific study, the outside facility needed to manually push the images to Balad. During our cycle, we installed a program to add studies on CD brought by patients to our local server. This permitted image transmittal on to LRMC as well as access to these images throughout the hospital. For this program to function, it was required that the images must be copied to CD as DICOM images. Constant reminders to assure this occurs were required.

Reading workstations are in Radiology as well as in the ER. There were also access links on personal computers in the surgery, ICU, and ward areas. When we moved to the new facility, we placed high-resolution color monitors in each of four operating rooms.

We constantly pushed for more bandwidth in the Area of Operations (AOR) to speed up image transfers in the AOR. In addition, we obtained a backup MedWeb Server, faster network routers and cabling, and more network support. A theater-wide contact sheet is on file in radiology. This was needed to communicate early with all theater radiologists to enhance and streamline operations and make upgrading the MedWeb more seamless and efficient.

Patients received from outside facilities often arrived with CDs with their images. At times, the CDs were not functional or they were not made. The ability through the web to pull and view images through teleradiology from Baghdad is theoretically available, but the poor bandwidth (slow transmission) and poor reliability of the connection (related most likely to security firewalls) continued to be problems during our rotation and past deployments.

There were two C-Arms owned, operated and maintained by the operating room. Although not our responsibility, some familiarity with the equipment is prudent since radiology is our profession and some will call upon us for help/advice. There were times when extra knowledge on these imaging resources (including US owned by other departments) was life-saving.

Myelogram contrast was available for occasional CT myelograms. Omnipaque 180 or Isoview 200M was ordered for safety and flexibility for adult and pediatric applications. Gastroview and barium were available with the C-Arms, our only fluoroscopy.

2.3.3 RIS/HIS

All trauma patients had their radiology results recorded by the radiologist into the Joint Patient Tracking System (JPTA), and the system has worked well. However, no system existed to record all inpatient/outpatient imaging results. Exam results are most often recorded on paper and delivered to the clinician. These written reports are sometimes lost and at times did not arrive at the patient's destination at the clinic, on the ward, or in the ICU. Verbal communication of results was commonplace, however, text reports were available in JPTA. If one radiologist did not have record of prior reads, we had to re-read an entire study to render information to the clinicians, especially before transport.

Although the system was not perfect, it was acceptable in the deployed environment. I would type the JPTA notes after the trauma cases are managed, and any other ER findings are communicated, provided urgent ICU images are also communicated to the docs/nurses. The JPTA notes on combat casualties were completed before outpatients are read.

MedWeb upgrade for electronic reporting with voice recognition package was installed. I was able to upload select CT images and compressed CT movie files into JPTA as an attachment that could be read anywhere in the AOR and CONUS, but the process was time consuming. The important thing was proof of concept. There will be more discussion on teleradiology, RIS/HIS later in this book.

The radiologists provided daily (8 a.m.) radiology rounds for the ICU team. This time allows the ICU team to review patient imaging exams and plan their daily treatments. The input from the providers was very helpful in understanding the severity of the casualty's status and maximized our ability to provide timely and more accurate interpretations.

2.4 Hospital Resources/Staffing

The 332nd Medical Group had about 40 Air Force providers to include Nurse Practitioners and Physician Assistants in addition to MDs and DOs. Since we were the only head and neck team in Iraq, we had five Head/Neck Team Providers to include two neurosurgeons, an ENT/maxillofacial surgeon, and an ophthalmologist. Two of our techs were dedicated to the head and neck team. There were also 24 Army Support Staff (OR staff/Nursing) with three Marines and one Navy support staff. The hospital had several interpreters available on a 24/7 basis.

2.5 Summary

This chapter provided an overview of the deployed combat hospital system in the military and capability/resources of each with a focus on the Level 3 facility. Some terminology has been introduced that will be seen again in following chapters.

2.6 Our Combat Radiology Department Library

Books purchased over the years for the radiologist reading room include the following:

Bone & Joint Imaging, 2nd Ed, Resnick
Caffey's Pediatric Diagnositic Imaging, 10th Ed, Kuhn, Slovis, & Haller
Computed Tomography: Physical Principles, Clinical Applications, & Quality pi Control, Seeram
Diagnostic Imaging: Head & Neck, Harnsberger
Fundamentals of Body CT, 3rd Ed, Webb, Brant, & Major
Fundamentals of Diagnostic Radiology, 2nd Ed, Brant & Helms
Genitourinary Radiology Requisites, 2nd Ed, Zagoria
Handbook of Interventional Radiologic Procedures, 3rd Ed, Kandarpa & Aruny
Helical (Spiral) Computed Tomography: A Practical Approach to Clinical Protocols, Silverman
Imaging in Trauma and Critical Care, Dr. Stu Mirvis
Keats Normal Variants
Neuroradiology Requisites, 2nd Ed, Grossman & Yousem
Radiology of Skeletal Trauma, 3rd Ed, Rogers
Ultrasound Requisites, 2nd Ed, Middleton, Kurtz, & Hertzberg

References

1. Curfman R. Temporary hospital finds permanent place in history. http://www.af.mil/news/story.asp?id=123092683 Accessed 15 August, 2009.
2. Folio LR. Challenges of Moving a Radiology Department during Combat Operations. Military Medical Technology. 22 Oct 2007, 11(7).
3. Tegtmeier E. R.T.s in Combat. Radiologic Technology. September/October 2007, 79(1): 1–2.
4. Mirvis S. Use of total body digital radiography (Statscan) for acute trauma imaging: preliminary experience in comparison with traditional computed tomography. 27 Nov 2005. Available at (accessed 24 August 2009): http://rsna2005.rsna.org/rsna2005/V2005/conference/event_display.cfm?em_id=4414276.
5. Beningfield S. Report on a new type of trauma full-body digital X-ray machine. Emergency Radiology 2003, 10:23–29.

Chapter 3
Blast and Ballistics: Types, Background, Terminology

Keywords IED · V-IED · EFP · RPG · Shrapnel · Fragment, Projectile, Missile · Ballistics, missile precession · Rifling, spinning · Wound ballistics, tumbling · Temporary, permanent wound cavity · Penetrating · Perforation · Missile embolus · Keyhole pattern

3.1 Introduction

Many combat casualties are victims of explosives, resulting in catastrophic polytrauma with multiple types of injuries. Terrorists attack in an attempt to drain resources, injuring many, with grueling psychological effects to help get their message across. Blast injuries are not as unique to battle as we would hope, however, as they are unfortunately becoming more common worldwide outside the battlefield environment. Familiarity with imaging manifestations of blast injuries, for example, is paramount no matter the setting, country, or location. Disasters, explosions, and shootings can happen in all types of settings and can occur anywhere. Some example cases of blast and ballistic injury are highlighted to illustrate our experiences in imaging findings and surgical follow-up in combat casualties.

3.2 Types of Explosives and Types of Resultant Blast Injuries

Few providers have had the opportunity to gain experience diagnosing and treating those severely injured from blast or high-velocity missiles. Most injuries in Iraq have been due Improvised Explosive Devices (IED). With explosions becoming more common in civilian settings to include the United States, understanding types and effects of blast injury can familiarize the radiologist and result in increased detection of imaging findings for optimal diagnosis, prognosis, and treatment options.

There are several types of explosive ordinance seen in modern combat worthy of discussing.

IED: Improvised Explosive Device that is home-made from everyday materials. The harmful projectiles include anything from paperclips and spent bullet shells to automobile parts (especially when the car is part of the bomb).

VB-IED: Vehicle-Borne Improvised Explosive Device: Essentially an IED that is placed in a vehicle.

RPG: Rocket Powered Grenade: a grenade that is shot from a rocket to explode on impact of a human, group, or structure to inflict damage.

EFP: Explosive Formed Penetrator: a tubular container capped with concave copper plates that project the plate by mechanics of reversal of the concavity to a convexity, providing additional thrust during the explosion. See Fig. 3.1 for sequential photos of a controlled detonation of VB-EFP that acted also like an IED in that the car parts acted as projectiles. These images should show how these homemade explosive devices can be devastating.

Example cases are included that highlight some of these properties and medical effects and imaging findings in casualties suffering from blast injuries. A brief description of medical blast effects is in order. There are four types of blast injury depending on proximity, severity, type of explosive, and surrounding environment [1, 2]:

Primary: Blast wave: hollow organs essentially burst due to overpressure
Secondary: Debris vs. body (most common, IED, other blasts)
Tertiary: Body thrown against hard objects (walls, objects)
Quaternary (or miscellaneous): Fire, smoke, crushing

Basically, primary blast injury comes from a wave of blast overpressure compressing the body and hollow air-filled organs; secondary injury results from flying debris and projectiles that have ballistic properties; tertiary injury happens when the patient's body becomes the flying object and collides with other objects (walls, vehicles, etc). Quaternary (sometimes referred to as miscellaneous) injury comes from burns from the blast heat or inhalation of gases and smoke released in the explosion. Many casualties have a combination of these injury types.

There was recently a case reported that demonstrated colon perforation from the primary blast wave [3]. We have seen other primary blast effects to include lung (Blast Lung Injury or BLI). Although described for years, BLI has a lot to be discovered, however, has been shown to be a major cause of immediate death at the scene of terrorist bombing attacks [4]. Work is underway to stage severity by CT findings of BLI at Walter Reed Army Medical Center. A spectrum of blast lung injuries with proposed mechanisms will be shown in the chest imaging chapter.

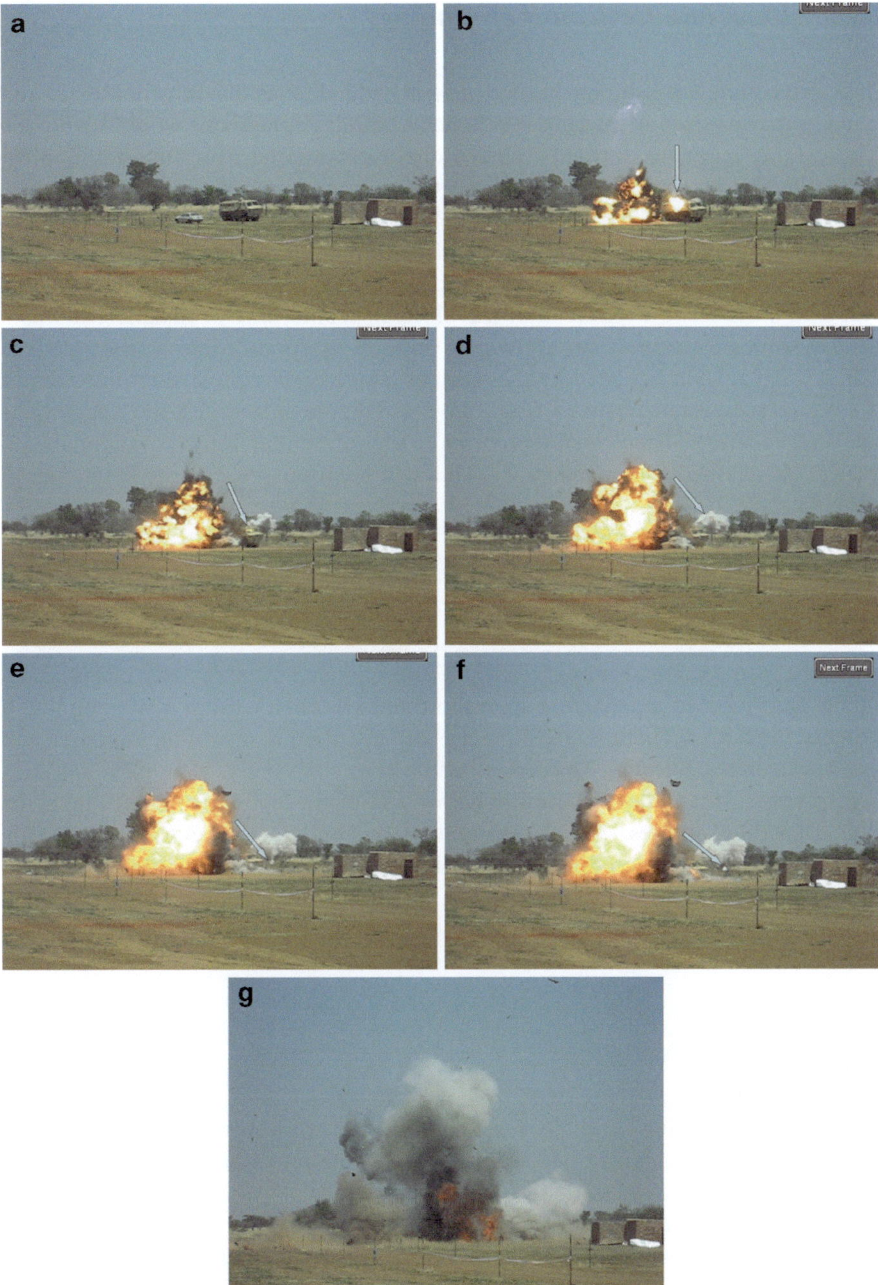

Fig. 3.1 These sequential photos demonstrate the destructive nature of an EFP. The armored vehicle was penetrated by the EFB placed into the adjacent small car. The effects of the copper plate (initial burning on entrance, burning copper in drivers compartment, smoke on exit, and resultant ash debris on exit) are seen by the arrow in each of the sequences. Photos by Dr. Les Folio

3.2.1 Blast and Ballistic Terminology

There are unique terms in the science of blast and ballistics that may not be familiar to many radiologists. Mastering this lexicon before deployment would be prudent since trauma surgeons and experienced deployers will be using this terminology regularly. For example, some still use the term "Shrapnel" however, that is a specific term reserved for the now obsolete artillery round developed by Henry Shrapnel, a young British Officer, at the end of the eighteenth century. This Shrapnel Shell, also called "case-shot" or "canister," was a metal canister filled with lead balls set to explode after traveling a specific time or distance. It was in use by Armies for more than 100 years, and fell essentially into disuse in World War I in 1915 when replaced by the more effective high explosive artillery rounds [5]. We refer to retained metal from blasts as fragments and describe their shape, size, and location. There is research underway at Walter Reed to automatically localize all retained fragments in 3D. This will be discussed in more detail later in this book.

3.2.2 Ballistics

Bullets spin on own axis (like a spinning football) when exiting a weapon due to rifling of the barrel. There is slight precession or wobbling that often increases with distance from the weapon. Once a projectile enters the body, it tumbles and most often reverses orientation where the heavy end of the bullet eventually takes the lead. This often causes the tapered end of the bullet to face back toward the direction the bullet entered. High-velocity firearms generally create the greatest amount of trauma, however, size, shape, and consistency of the bullet (jacketed, hollow point, etc.) have influence over the extent of the wound.

3.2.3 Wound Ballistics

The terms "penetrating" and "perforating" injuries, while very different, are often confused for one another. In penetrating injuries, the projectiles (or missiles) enter the body and do not exit, while in perforating injuries, they enter and exit; through and through injuries essentially. In addition, bullets, associated fragments, and blast debris may enter a vessel and embolize to the lungs or brain. This is sometimes referred to as missile embolus, and is well-documented [6–8]. Once intravascular, any migration of the bullet/fragment will be influenced by position, respiratory motion, blood flow, and gravitational forces [9, 10]. Operative manipulation alone has been described in causing fragment migration [11]. One recent documentation of missile embolus was nicely illustrated by Andrews et al. [12]. This fragment from an AK 47 round was documented with regard to the knee, then was not seen on follow-up knee plain images, then seen on a follow-up CXR that was clear hours earlier.

3.2.4 Wound Cavities

The permanent wound cavity is the damage done directly by the projectile along its immediate path. There is also a temporary wound cavity, caused by pressure waves created by and following the projectile as it passes through surrounding tissues separated from the bullet. The temporary cavity is generally larger than the diameter of the bullet [13]. This temporary wound cavity is created by deformation of tissue as it is displaced by the pressure wave. Some tissue stretch easily and are less vulnerable to damage by this mechanism, such as muscle. Other, more friable tissue, as in solid organs like liver or spleen, are more vulnerable to damage. Mechanisms of trauma are a result of crushing and stretching of tissues from the often tumbling projectile [14]. Figure 3.2 demonstrates a GSW to the chest that shows a laceration of the lung in the direct path of the bullet, with surrounding consolidation representing the local destruction of lung tissue and associated vasculature.

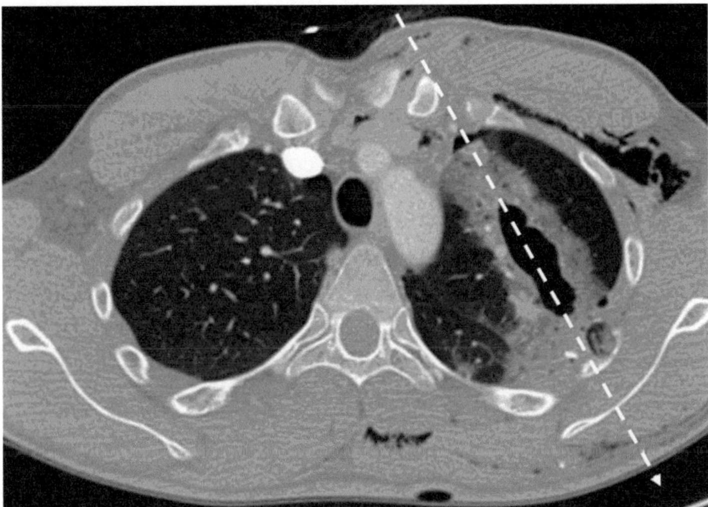

Fig. 3.2 This reformatted para-axial thorax CTA demonstrates the lung laceration representing the permanent cavity, and the surrounding consolidation representing contusion of the temporary cavity of the perforating tumbling projectile. C-Arm interoperative selective ICA angiogram with isolated CTA 3-D correlation (3B). Reprinted with permission from Military Medicine: International Journal of AMSUS

3.2.5   Even Number Guide

When a casualty suffers from multiple GSW, a basic guide may be helpful to account for all fragments based on wounds and imaging findings. The even number guide is based on the number entrance and exit wounds should be associated with number of fragments expected on imaging. This assumes GSWs without fragmentation and occasionally may work with blast fragments. Basically, the total number of bullets and wounds should be an even number [15]. The simplest example would be a penetrating GSW with an entrance and no exit. One entrance wound means one fragment should be expected on imaging (total of two, an even number). If a fragment is not seen on initial imaging, then more imaging may be necessary, even in remote anatomic regions. One reason for this is the possibility of a missile embolus just mentioned. Another example to highlight the even number guide would be a casualty with three entrance wounds and one exit wound. One would expect to find two bullets for a total of six – an even number. This may not seem necessary at first, however, with multiple GSW casualties, each with multiple GSWs, every tool to simplify matters can be more helpful than first realized.

There are some injuries that have characteristic imaging patterns that help determine prognosis, cause and manner of death, and may help in analysis of incident. Later in this book I will present a case of a soldier wounded in Iraq with a gunshot wound to the skull exhibiting this characteristic keyhole fracture pattern on CT [16]. Tangential gunshot wounds to the skull were originally termed "keyhole fractures" by Spitz in 1980, and the mechanics involved in the creation of the defect were later described by Dixon in 1982 [17]. Keyhole fractures exhibit entrance and exit wound defects resulting from a projectile striking the cranium or long bones tangentially. The projectile's initial impact creates a circular entrance defect as the bullet strikes the outer table of bone, and a secondary fracture is created by bone fragments propagated from the initial point of impact [18]. External examination of the wound can therefore be confusing, manifesting signs of both entrance and exit type trauma [19]. This is important information for the radiologist to provide to the ED doc urgently since the wound can seem trivial on clinical inspection. Awareness of the mechanics behind tangential gunshot wounds can help classify the type of injury and the associated trauma incurred by the patient. CT is important in the medical work up of tangential gunshot wounds as it can show the keyhole fracture of the cranium as well as any bone fragments within the calvarium.

3.3   Summary

Imaging in blast and ballistic injuries can be puzzling if not prepared or familiar with findings and/or terminology. This chapter introduced some basic lexicon to help orient the radiologist to the lingo used in combat hospitals and some busy trauma centers that see these types of injuries. Although blast injuries may not be common in most hospitals, familiarity with lessons learned in combat would be prudent for if and when a blast does occur. Even a basic understanding of blast properties and potential effects on the body can help the radiologist more effectively communicate with ED docs and trauma surgeons.

References

1. DePalma RG, Burris DG, Champion HR. Current concepts blast injuries. N Engl J Med. 2005 31 March,352(13):1335–1342.
2. Eastridge BJ. Things that go boom: injuries from explosives. J Trauma. 2007,62(6 Suppl):S38.
3. Bounovas A, Perente S, Laftsidis P, Polychronidis A, Simopoulos C. Perforation of the colon from the primary blast effect of an extraperitoneal shotgun injury: case report. Mil Med. 2007 Mar,172(3):327–8.
4. Avidan V, Hersch M, Armon Y et al. Blast lung injury: clinical manifestations, treatment, and outcome. Am J Surg. 2005,190:927–31.
5. Rich N, Burris D. Letters to the editor. J Trauma. 2006 Oct,61(4):1024.
6. Bland EF, Beebe GW. Missiles in the heart: a twenty-year follow-up report of World War II cases. N Engl J Med. 1966 May,274(19):1039–46.
7. Bernini CO, Junqueira AR Jr, Horita LT et al. Pulmonary embolism from gunshot missiles. Surg Gynecol Obstet. 1983 May,156(5):615–9.
8. Nehme AE. Intracranial bullet migrating to pulmonary artery. J Trauma. 1980 Apr,20(4):344–6.
9. Singer RL, Dangleben DA, Salim A, Kurek SJ, Shah KT, Goodreau JJ, Shaff DI, Szydlowski GW. Missile embolism to the pulmonary artery: case report and pitfalls of management. Ann Thorac Surg. 2003 Nov,76(5):1722–5.
10. Stephenson LW, Workman RB, Aldrete JS, Karp RB. Bullet emboli to the pulmonary artery: a report of 2 patients and review of the literature. Ann Thorac Surg. 1976 Apr,21(4):333–6.
11. Bertoldo U, Enrichens F, Comba A, Ghiselli G et al. Retrograde venous bullet embolism: a rare occurrence – case report and literature review. J Trauma. 2004 Jul,57(1):187–92.
12. Andrews C, Andrews K, Folio L. Venous fragment embolism to the pulmonary artery: a rare occurrence – case report and literature review of venous fragment embolization to the pulmonary artery. Mil Med. 2009 Sept,174(9):iv,v.
13. DiMaio MD, Vincent JM. 1999 Gunshot Wounds: Practical Aspects of Firearms, Ballistics, and Forensic Techniques, 2nd Edition. Boca Raton: CRC Press.
14. Fackler ML. Ballistic injury. Ann Emerg Med. 1986,15(12):1451–5.
15. Folio LR, McHugh, Hoffman M. The even number guide: a method for accounting for ballistic injuries. Radiol Technol. 2007 Jan/Feb,78(3):197–203.
16. Jackson AM, Searcey BK, Smirniotopoulos JG, Folio L. Keyhole fracture of the skull. Mil Med. 2008 Dec,173(12):xix–xx.
17. Spitz WU. 1980 Injury by gunfire: gunshot wounds. In: Spitz WU, Fisher RS, editors. Medicolegal Investigations of Death: Guidelines for the Application of Pathology to Crime Investigation. Springfield, IL: Charles C Thomas.
18. Dixon DS. Keyhole lesions in gunshot wounds to the skull and direction of fire. J Forensic Sci. 1982,27:555–6.
19. Berryman HE, Gunther WM. Keyhole defect production in tubular bone. J Forensic Sci. 2000 Mar,45(2):483–7.

Chapter 4
Introduction to Imaging of Penetrating/ Perforating Blast and Ballistic Injuries

Keywords NATO litter · Level 3 facility · Traua czar · Surgeon of the Day · Damage control surgery · Damage control imaging · CT Scout · Retriage · Protocolization · Surge/ Mass casualty

Diagnostic imaging in combat has many unique characteristics and situations that are briefly covered in this chapter. The diagnostic radiology mission is only a part of the complex system that needs to be understood. A team approach with integration with ED, OR, and ICU/ wards is imperative. Some of the unique aspects of combat radiology include the horrific nature of injuries, the multiplicity of severe trauma, and sheer number of injuries and casualties that can come at once. A common practice that may not be initially intuitive is diagnosing and treating regardless of "sides" in that we treat insurgents, prisoners, local nationals, Iraqi police, Military Working Dogs, children [1], and pregnant women with threat to life, limb, or eyesight.

The severity of battle injuries and necessity for immediate treatment relates to US trauma centers in some ways. However, in the haze of battle, resource limitations, physical and emotional fatigue, the intensity seen in a civilian facility simply cannot compare to that of a combat hospital. These limitations are somehow miraculously overcome thanks to the spirit, determination, and motivation of all hospital staff to do the right thing. We press on to the point of exhaustion, pass out (sleep), exercise and start each day all over again. There are no real weekends since we work every day; in fact, some refer to each day as Groundhog Day (like the movie, not 2 Feb). In the words of Colonel Masterson, our medical group commander in 2007, "everyday is an eternity, every month is a moment."

From an imaging perspective, for example, hypoperfusion complex and hypovolemia CT findings are enhanced (more periportal fluid, flatter IVC, enhanced, fluid filled small bowel, etc.). Casualties are often dehydrated and volume depleted and/or hypertonic to begin with from the extreme heat and protective gear. They also often have severe blood loss, and have been transported in a tight, hot environment such as a helicopter with hot air blowing in the open bay. Included in this chapter is a case of shock bowel/flat IVC as a radiographic surrogate for hypovolemia, hypoperfusion complex, and impending bowel ischemia.

When new hospital staff arrive in a deployed field hospital, they have three days to learn from the staff that are on their way out. Imagine changing out 95% of trauma level 1 hospital staff in three days while keeping operations at full capacity without limitation. This may be done a few times a year. It is truly amazing how people can be trained up in workflow and procedures in such a short period of time; somehow this seemingly complex event happens without fail or compromise in patient care. My most recent deployment to Iraq included an additional transition where we moved our entire trauma hospital from the original tent configuration to a hardened facility. With months of preparation, the actual move occurred in less than 90 min with continual care. In radiology, we had combat trauma patients being imaged in both hospitals at the same time with dual staff and split equipment [2].

Within a few weeks, the deployed providers are exposed to the near-overwhelming workload and are already blunted to the point that regularly called trauma codes with urgent patients massively wounded become seemingly routine. America can claim victory over the most successful recoverability of combat casualties in history with the highest rates of survivability, fastest transport, optimal body armor and protection, and the best technology.

4.1 Trauma Flow and Throughput of Casualties in a Deployed Combat Hospital

The most critical patients arrive by helicopter; however, patients also arrive by ambulance and walk in, and injured patients are often dropped off at the base gate from the local area. Urgent and priority litter patients are wheeled into the main emergency department from the helicopters using NATO litters (see Fig. 4.1). These litters have locks that turn into the "table" where the patient receives resuscitation and triage in the ER. Ambulatory and routine litters go to a separate section. See Fig. 4.2 showing how the NATO litter is being pushed by one OR tech in the tent facility.

The radiologist plays a key role in radiologic triage and protocolization. The radiologist and radiologic technologist respond as part of the primary trauma response team. There is at least one radiologist covering the department for trauma and critical care follow-up 24/7, as many US trauma centers now do. When many urgent casualties come at one time (a "surge"), the radiologist, ED doctor, and traumatologist (trauma czar) triage the imaging resources (techs, portables, CT's) since many casualties will have to wait for imaging during surges (e.g., 20–30 combat casualties at once). This radiologist/ traumatologist triage of imaging resources has been recommended in the past [3].

Like most trauma centers and emergency departments, the first imaging obtained on warfighters in combat hospitals is the CXR, and on occasion, the pelvis.

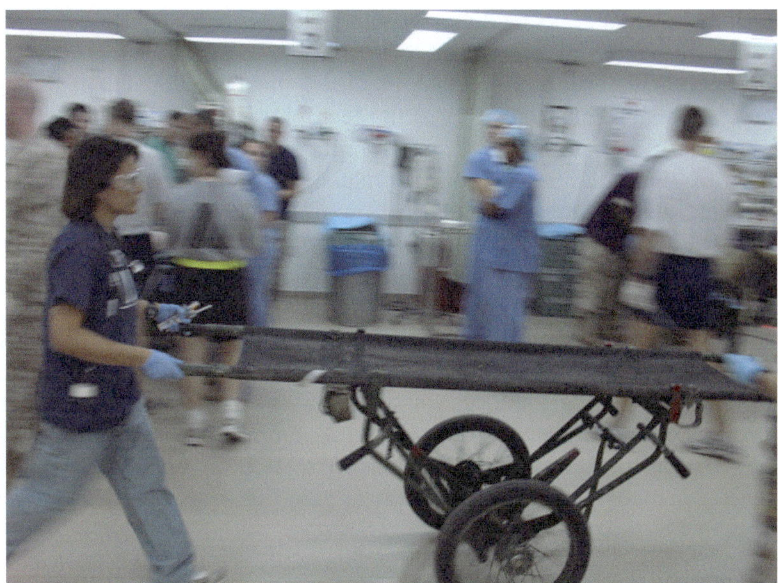

Fig. 4.1 The NATO litter is seen here in the ED of the new facility we moved into during our deployment

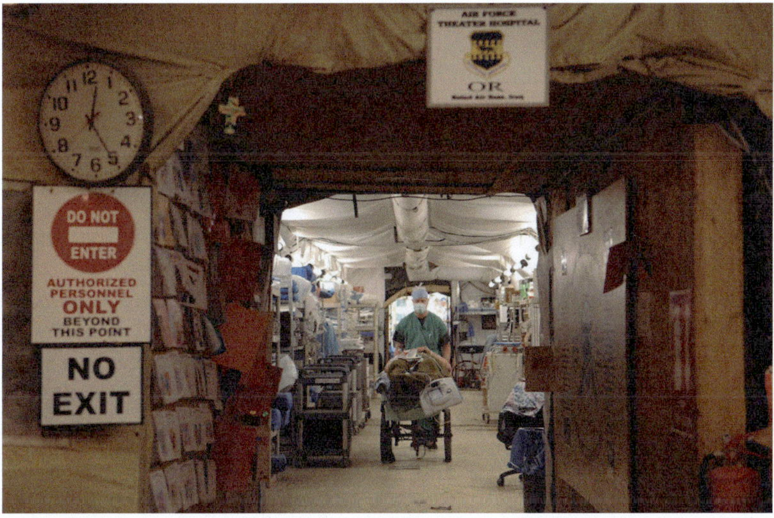

Fig. 4.2 This shows how the NATO litter can be pushed by one person, here in the tent facility OR

We rarely do lateral cervical spines in the extreme polytrauma encountered in combat since they will be getting a CT anyway. It must be kept in mind that most X-ray techs sent to combat are not CT techs, yet they must learn how to perform CTs in 3 days. Keeping the protocols simple and standard without much special sequences is key. Three technologists and a radiologist respond to every trauma code; one tech helps with movement and stabilization of the patient with a plate close by. When the patient is rolled to check the back for spinal deformity/tenderness, abrasions, and rectal tone, the tech places the CXR plate under that patient's chest. With multiple patients or during surges, techs watch to see which patient will be ready for a CXR next (typically happens at certain stabilization phases), what the radiologist is gathering by the SOD (Surgeon of the Day) and individual ER docs (one doc per patient), and who is ready next. If the patient needs pelvis X-ray, this is often done immediately after the CXR.

Similar to US trauma centers, imaging is integral in management within the golden hour(s). If the patient does not require immediate damage control surgery, or has a negative FAST (Focused Abdominal Sonography for Trauma), the patient goes to CT for either a PanScan (in blast, or injury distraction scenarios) or dedicated anatomical regions for isolated GSW. From there, surgical intervention is planned, avoided if no indication, then off to ICU. A positive FAST and/or deteriorating hemodynamic state may dictate going strait to the OR for definitive management and skip CT.

The FAST is done by the ED doctors in combat hospitals and sensitive enough to help make the decision to go strait to the OR and save the CT resources for others. It is especially useful for level 2 facilities (hospitals without CT). It does not take long – a few days on the combat trauma scene – to really appreciate the usefulness of FAST. During our deployment, the emergency department evaluated E-FAST (Extended FAST) [4].

A new frame of treatment has evolved with battlefield medicine called damage control surgery [5], where emergent surgery is done to control bleeding and treat the most amount of casualties [6], and deployed radiology needs to parallel this thinking to be effective in combat. Regarding stabilization and assessment in the combat ER, one needs to understand the concept of damage control surgery. Rather than Airway Breathing Circulation, managing severe battle injuries in the field and in the combat ER requires a backward approach to this concept in that Circulation needs to be controlled first in the ED, then Breathing, then Airway.

Chest and Pelvis plain CR are often done before CT (or going to the OR), and C-Spine is done as part of the PanScan. The chest X-ray CR (Computed Radiography) plate is placed behind the patient when rolled up to check the spine and rectal tone. The chest (and pelvis, when obtained) CR plates are also run first as to not slow down the resulting of these to the ER docs and surgeons. For casualties going direct to the OR, extremities may be taken in a higher priority on those patients.

There are several instances in this book where the CXR, shot through lateral C-spine and pelvis plain X-rays, were not obtained in the emergency room. Since the X-ray technologist was often the limiting resource, time could be saved and resources allocated to allow technologists to get the portable CXRs and pelvis X-rays on casualties going directly to the OR. In our experience, we found that the CT scouts (AP and lateral) of the chest were fast and adequate in lieu of the portable CXRs in the ED. If we were getting the CT anyway on hemodynamic stable casualties, the CT scout view often sufficed for the CXR since we were going to obtain more detail on the CT findings minutes after that. We also felt that the CT scouts were faster, more efficient to reallocate our technologist resources, and of better quality of care overall.

When it comes to interpretation of massive volumes of CT images, extremities, ICU chests, there are methods to the madness. In combat, many surgeries are performed at the same time, with surgical specialists operating on any available surface. When we were in the tent facilities, the isoshelter operating rooms would often have multiple surgeries going on at time on each patient (i.e. neurosurgeon at the head of the patient, urologist in the abdomen and an orthopedic surgeon at the legs). I have seen up to seven surgeries being done at once in one isoshelter operating room. Keeping this in mind, an order of procedures is tailored to each patient, depending on severity and nature of the various injuries, and the tailoring of the CT needs to parallel this requirement. Deviating from an established routine is the only consistent thing in the fog of combat imaging. The following "damage control imaging" helped me.

4.2 Damage Control Imaging

While deployed, I developed a more streamlined imaging request form in concert with the ED and the trauma czar (representing all trauma surgeons) to guide ordering of studies and where to write results in a standard fashion (see Fig. 4.3). This change simplified the ordering by ED staff, made filling out by radiologists more efficient, and ease of finding the results for medical staff. A "primary survey" of the entire body is often helpful using the AP, and lateral scout provides an overview of metallic fragments, CXR, fractures, etc. A quick view bone windows of the head is useful looking for major fracture, soft tissue indicators of trauma, and/or metal. This is followed by brain windows in search for hematomas, cistern effacement, or midline shift. If there is time, viewing C spine keeps a methodical head to toe pattern, however, this is more often interrupted by trauma surgeons wanting to know if they need to operate (presence of lung or abdominal fluid, organ damage or penetration of peritoneum or retroperitoneum). The C Spine can be reviewed while the patient is being transported to the OR.

I found myself screening quickly through the Chest Abdomen and Pelvis (C/A/P), with a combination lung/ bone window (for example: W2000 L20) through whole body for a big picture of fragments, trajectories, free air, or other significant evidence of intraperitoneal compromise. This allowed me to get the most life threatening injury findings to the surgeons that needed to plan for immediate life saving surgery.

In combat hospitals, the focus falls on efficient throughput, detecting lung lacerations or hemothoraxes, recognizing vessel contrast extravasation, diagnosing free air in non-dependent abdomen and locating major displaced fractures of the spine or pelvis. All, of course, in as many patients as possible, in the shortest

Radiology Form: Trauma/ Surge/ MassCal

332 EMDG   AGE:____

Radiology Phone 443-8527

US Name, trauma # or TCN/LN #

NOTE: for mass casualty, can substitute Trauma Number only for Name and SSN

Rad Tech Name: **Time of Exam:**   SS#   _____ - ___ - _____

Location:	ER 443-8513						Date:	Day	Month	Year
From:	Field	10th	FOB:			Other:				

History: (Circle one)   IED Mortar Gunshot MVA EET Central Line NG/OG Tube

Provider/ER staff: Please circle requested exams:

X-Ray Exams			Results
CXR		CXR by CT Scout	
		Pelvis	
Other (eg. KUB, Lat C Spine)			
RT	LT	SHOULDER	
RT	LT	HUMERUS	
RT	LT	ELBOW	
RT	LT	FOREARM	
RT	LT	WRIST	
RT	LT	HAND	
RT	LT	FEMUR	
RT	LT	KNEE	
RT	LT	TIB/FIB	
RT	LT	ANKLE	
RT	LT	FOOT	

CT Exams

		Negative	Positive (if positive, fill out below findings)			
PanScan	Head	Missile track? No Yes	Unilobar ?: No Yes (___ lobe)	Bihemispheric? No Yes	Multilobar? No Yes	Transventricular? No Yes
		CT findings c/w elevated ICP? No Yes		Sulci? Effaced Patent	Cisterns? Patent Effaced	Midline shift? No Yes (_____ mm)
		Hemorrhage? No Yes	Intraparenchymal hemorrhage? No Yes ___ x ___ x ___ mm ___ lobe		Cisternal? SAH? IVH?	Extra-axial? No Yes (__ DH)
		Pneumocephalus? No Yes		Other:		
	C-Spine					
	Chest					
	Abdomen					
	Pelvis					
	CTA COW					
	CT Face					
	CTA Carotids					
	CTA Chest					
	Other (eg. T+L Spine)					

Findings Continued on Back if Checked ▢

Additional forms available on t drive under T:\Radiology\Admin Files\Forms

Updated 21 July 2007

FIRMR (41 CRF) 101-11.806-8

Fig. 4.3 The streamlined form for ordering imaging studies and reporting in a standard fashion. Knowing where to look for reports on body regions and types of studies was proven helpful during our deployment

amount of time. Similar experiences from other radiologists have led to the creation of software to allow for a single trauma window to view lung, soft tissues and bone all in one sweep. Research is underway to study this universal trauma window at Walter Reed Army Medical Center.

After surgical disposition is determined on the current wave of patients, it is a good time to review the scans in more detail for a definitive final interpretation, or "secondary survey." Jotting findings down on the streamlined form acts as a good template for entering into the EMR at a later time. Many times the data entry is at the end of a shift when there is relief by the next radiologist shift. By the way, all this is going on while helicopters continue to land two, three, or four at a time while the base is under attack. The radiologists are also back and forth to the trauma bays providing updated answers as we discover them, as well as trips to the ORs, ICU on traumas evaluated and treated earlier. The noise of the helicopters and staff speaking loudly above that baseline noise in tents, heat, etc. can compound the stress and pressures of knowing your responsibility to help save life, limb, and eyesight in the fog of war.

In a mass casualty or disaster, more hospital staff is called in from their rest, however, if prolonged, rest–work cycles as well as continued supply stocking, distribution, and modified roles and responsibilities are taken into consideration. The work cycle is a fast-paced, all-production operation for 120–180 days. One learns new ways of doing business – but one must know one's own field as a baseline: this is no place for brushing up on trauma skills. One must also be creative when seeming overwhelmed. We would often put our waiting outpatients to work (that were able) as they realized they would be tended to faster by helping radiology or ER staff (manpower, getting water for techs, communicating by running, etc.). Walkie-talkie triage works in combat; patients bending over in pain or unable to walk take higher priority over those who can walk and help.

4.3 Unique Radiology Protocolization in Extreme Trauma

See Fig. 4.4 for a quick-reference spreadsheet for trauma CT protocols that evolved for our deployed radiology department. The one page/quick reference highlights the combined studies and shortcuts that we could tailor to each patient. The CT of head without contrast, cervical spine, chest, abdomen, and pelvis with contrast (PanScan, not dissimilar to "ShanScan" commonly refered to at Baltimore Shock Trauma, thanks to Dr. Shanmuganathan) is very common and almost universally done in blast injuries. It was not a policy to do a PanScan on every patient coming to the ER, as this would not be time or radiation/contrast dose effective. This spreadsheet is available on the Air Force Readiness Skills Verification webpage, the online course for deploying radiologists mentioned earlier.

For penetrating injuries potentially involving the subclavian arteries or other great vessels near the neck and chest, the arm opposite the penetration is injected. This minimizes beam hardening artifact from contrast concentration in the brachiocephalics near the potential damaged vessels.

For pelvic fracture stability determination, we commonly reconstruct the pelvis from the PanScan in transparent 3D to provide a pseudo X-ray inlet/ outlet view, without spending time to take plain radiographs. This allows for diagnosing with

	PROTOCOL	INDICATIONS	Slice	Start-end	IV Contrast	Delay (sec)	Filter	REC 1	REC 2"	MPR	Send to EBV	Send to Medweb
1				Dr. Folio's Quick-Reference Trauma CT PROTOCOLS - Phillips Brialliance CT 2.0 16 MDCT								
3	PanScan (see each body part protocol below), consider doing CT scout CXR, if okay with ER, OR											
4	Basic:	Blast protocol		Head with bone recon, C-spine with Sag/cor recon, C/A/P with bone recon Sag/cor of spine							All	Brain, Spine Sag/Co
5	With Face:	With facial injury/ penetration		Basic (above) with Face with soft tissue recon							All	Basic, add face
6	With CTA Carotids:	Penetrating injury		Basic with CTA carotids with 3mm soft tissue recons, Sag/Cor of soft tissue recons (C-spine)								Basic, with CTA 3/3
7	With Face and CTA Carotids			Basic (above), add head with bone recon (soft?), face with soft tissue recon (bone?), CTA from above								
9	CTA											
10	CTA neck (carotids)	Penetrating injury neck, shoulder	1/0.5	Arch-Skull top	100ml @ 4ml/sec	15-20 or BT	Smooth (A)	3/3		Sag/Cor Cspine	1/1.5	3/3
11	CTA Aorta		2/1	Aorta-iliac bifr	100ml @ 4ml/sec	25s or BT	Smooth (A)	None		None	All	All
12	Aorta runoff		2/1	Ren art-pop	100ml @ 4ml/sec	25s or BT	Smooth (A)	None		None	All	All
13	CTA Chest (PE)		3/1.5	Apex-top kidneys	100ml @ 4ml/sec	18 or BT MPA	Smooth (A) 5/5 LungL					
14	Lower Extremity		5/2.5			BT						
16	Head neck											
17	Head (axial)	Trauma, blast, GSW, do Csp	4.5/4.5	Skull top-base	Non-con		Brain sharp	Bone		None	Brain/bone	Brain/bone
18	C-Spine	If suspect C-spine/ distracting inj	1/1.0	Skull base-T2	Non-con		Bone (D)	2/2 B ?		Sag/Cor	All	2/2 B Sag/Cor
19	Face	Can combine w face/ CTA	1/1.0	Top front-btm mand	None			3/1.5 S	3/3 B		all	3/1.5B, Cor MPR
20	Orbits			Top front-btm max	None							
21	Coronal Sinus		3	Ant to frontal-eth	None		bone			None	All	All
22	Head (helical)	Trauma, blast	5/5	Skull top-base	Non-con		Brain sharp	Bone		None	All	All
23	Head without/ with	Rule out tumor, mass, met	4.5/4.5	Skull top-base	75ml 2.5ml/s	3 min	Brain sharp				All	All
24	C-Spine w disk sp	If suspect disk injury	1/1.0	Skull base-T2	Non-con		Bone (D)	2/2 B	2.2 Smo	Sag/Cor	All	2/2 B Sag/Cor
25	Neck Soft Tissues		3/1.5	COW-Arch	100ml @ 3ml/sec	30s		3/3 ST		None	All	All
26	CT Myelogram											
28	Body											
29	C/A/P		5/5.0	Apex-Isc Tub	100ml @ 3ml/sec	50	Soft T	3/1.5(B,D)		Sag/Cor Sp B	All	ST C/A/P, Sag/Cor Sp
30	Chest		5/5.0	Apex-top kidneys	100ml @ 3ml/sec	30	Soft Tiss	Lung (L)		None	All	All
31	High Res Chest	See protocol book	1/0.5	Apex-top kidneys	Non		Soft Tiss	Lung (L)		None	All	See protocol book
32	A/P	GSW, Isolated blast	5/5.0	Diaph-Isc Tub	100ml @ 3ml/sec	60-70	Soft T(B)	3/1.5(B,D)		Sag/Cor Sp	All	5/5 A/P, Sag/Cor Sp
33	Liver 3 phase			Diaph-through liver	150ml @ 4ml/sec	Non, 28, 60	Soft T(B)	None		None	All	All
34	Pancreas 3 phase			Diaph-through liver	150ml @ 4ml/sec	Non, 42, 60	Soft T(B)	None		None	All	All
36	MSK											
37	T-Spine	R/O fracture, displaced or open	3/1.5	C7-L2	Non-con		Bone (D)	None		Sag/Cor	All	All
38	T-Spine w/disk sp		1/1.0	C7-L2	Non-con		Bone (D)	2/2 B	2/2 Smth	Sag/Cor of Stis	All	T Sp(B), Sag/cor ST
39	L-Spine		3/1.5	T11-S1	Non-con		Bone (D)	None		Sag/Cor	All	All

Pop-up note (over cells B11–B16): For CT venography to rule out DVT: use 370, 100 cc at 2cc/min, can use tracker at high threshold and watch for contrast in veins

Trauma

Fig. 4.4 This one page Excel spreadsheet carried all the protocol information developed by previous radiologists and radiologic technologists. It is conditionally formatted with pop-up information to provide more information in a condensed, easy to refer to format

SSN	Name	From:	Injuries	□ H/P □ 3899 # Proc
□ CT Head □ CT C/A/P □ Spine □ CTA □ Other		□ IED □ VBIED □ GSW □ BLUNT		
SSN	Name	From:	Injuries	□ H/P □ 3899 # Proc
□ CT Head □ CT C/A/P □ Spine □ CTA □ Other		□ IED □ VBIED □ GSW □ BLUNT		
SSN	Name	From:	Injuries	□ H/P □ 3899 # Proc
□ CT Head □ CT C/A/P □ Spine □ CTA □ Other		□ IED □ VBIED □ GSW □ BLUNT		
SSN	Name	From:	Injuries	□ H/P □ 3899 # Proc
□ CT Head □ CT C/A/P □ Spine □ CTA □ Other		□ IED □ VBIED □ GSW □ BLUNT		

Fig. 4.5 The SOD (Surgeon of the Day) sheet was used by the lead trauma surgeon for a shift to keep track of casualties for personal use and handing off to the next SOD. I used these myself to keep track of casualties and retriage to CT and to OR based on assessments and CT findings. This would provide a checklist of all patients I would need to provide textual reports for our medical record, and which ones that may need additional attention

familiar views for typing pelvic fracture stability and management. The value of instant coronal, sagittal, 3-D, MIP, and vessel tracking is paramount in combat trauma imaging. This has been described elsewhere [9] and within this text, and will be illustrated here, as combat injuries are no exception.

I also used an SOD sheet (see Fig. 4.5) for tracking small surges (mini-mass casualties that we got regularly). It would allow me to keep track of which patient was where with what major mechanism of injury, what CT we were going to do, and where. It is optimal to keep the least hemodynamically stable patient in the ED CT scanner since it is closer to the most ACLS providers. In addition, all radiologists in the Air Force are ACLS certified/current. One hospital is trying a method of re-triaging to CT vs. OR vs. ICU using Air Traffic Control (ATC) methods. Hoskins, et al studied the potential for using ATC in field exercises [10] based on our experiences in Iraq. See Fig. 4.6 for how we tested this retriaging tool in a field exercise with our university.

Blast injuries deserve special attention since we are still researching effects of blast, especially primary effects [11]. These principles will be discussed further in the next chapter. Distracting multiple injuries, high adrenaline of battle in young athletic military types, and high doses of morphine on board dictated a lower threshold for CT from head to pubes. Like anywhere else, CT is pivotal in poly-trauma for surgical triage, planning, and guidance. The epidemiological principles of pre and posttest probability and prevalence of "disease" should be kept in mind in that in our patient population, there is 80–90% trauma, whereas in many military medical centers in the US, it may be only 10–20%.

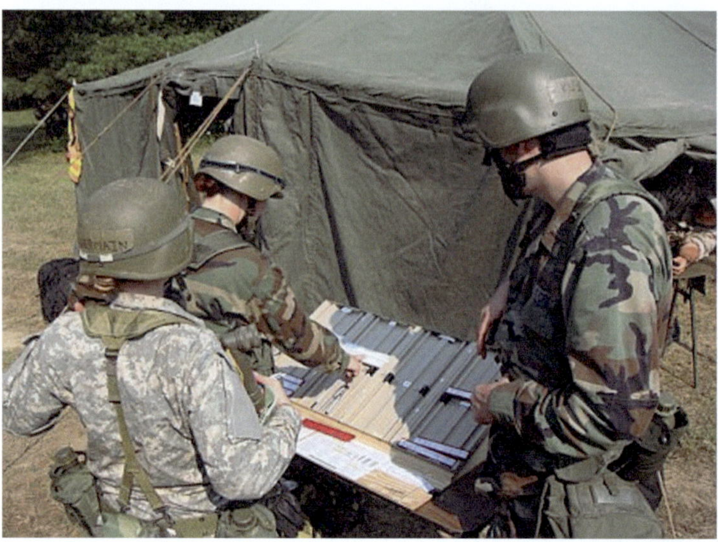

Fig. 4.6 This photo was taken during field exercises while testing Air Traffic Control methods to keep track of casualties. This method was more efficient and accurate in tracking casualties and now being evaluated in civilian trauma centers and a combat hospital

References

1. McGuigan R, Spinella PC, Beekley A, Sebesta J, Perkins J, Grathwohl K, Azarow K. Pediatric trauma: experience of a combat support hospital in Iraq. J Pediatr Surg. 2007 Jan,42 (1):207–10.
2. Folio LR. Challenges of moving a radiology department during combat operations. Mil Med Technol. 22 Oct 2007,11(7). Also available at: http://www.military-medical-technology.com/mmt-home/162-mmt-2007-volume-11-issue-7/1417-the-move-from-tent-city.html (accessed July 2010).
3. Mirvis S, Shanmuganathan K. Imaging in Trauma and Critical Care, 2nd Edition, 2003. Saunders, Philadelphia, PA.
4. Wilkerson RG, Stone MB. Sensitivity of bedside ultrasound and supine anteroposterior chest radiographs for the identification of pneumothorax after blunt trauma. Acad Emerg Med. 2010 Jan,17(1):11–7.
5. Ingari JV, Powell E. Civilian and detainee orthopaedic surgical care at an Air Force theater hospital. Tech Hand Up Extrem Surg. 2007 Jun,11(2):130–4.
6. Sambasivan CN, Schreiber MA. Emerging therapies in traumatic hemorrhage control. Curr Opin Crit Care. 2009 Dec,15(6):560–8.
7. Choi R, Folio L. U.S. Patent Application No. 12/175,308. Multi-Grayscale Overlay Window.
8. Fischer T, Folio L. Universal Trauma Window; A combined Window for Preliminary Review of Mass Casualties. American Society of Emergency Radiologists. October 2009.
9. Harcke HT, Levy AD, Getz JM, Robinson SR. MDCT analysis of projectile injury in forensic investigation. AJR Am J Roentgenol. 2008 Feb,190(2):W106–11.
10. Hoskins J, Graham R, Robinson D, Lutz C, Folio L. Repurposing air traffic control to track combat casualties more effectively. J Am Coll Surg. 2009 June,208(6):1001–8.
11. Tsokos M, Paulsen F, Petri S, et.al. Histologic, immunohistochemical, and ultrastructural findings in human blast lung injury. Am J Respir Crit Care Med. 2003,168:549–5.

Chapter 5
Significant Medical Advances on the Battlefield and the Changing Roles of Imaging

Keywords Combat application tourniquet · Tactical combat casualty care · Casualty evacuation · Medical evacuation · Air evacuation · Extended focused abdominal sonography in trauma · Anatomic positioning system · Trajectory analysis · Decision support tools · Health vault · Universal trauma window

5.1   Record Survival Rates of Combat Casualties

American and coalition forces can claim one overwhelming victory in recent conflicts: the highest survival rate of combat casualties in history. Approximately 98% of all casualties brought to our facility survived, a higher percentage than ever before in prior wars. Some of the most obvious contributions to these record survival rates are due to advances such as the Combat Application Tourniquet (CAT) and its clear indications from TCCC (Tactical Combat Casualty Care). Other major contributors to heroic survival success is clearly due to improved helicopter casualty and medical evacuation from the front lines to the many combat hospitals. In addition, Air Force air evacuation out of war zone to the upper echelons of care is described earlier in this book. Myself and others believe advanced imaging techniques and applications, some discussed here, have also significantly contributed to these record survival rates.

An example of heroic performance of medical professionals in battle conditions is best exemplified by the helicopter combat medics that rescue the combat casualties from the point of injury. While often under fire, these medics and helicopter crews bring casualties on battlefield to advanced imaging and surgical capability in record time, often in minutes within initial injury. When active shooting and bombing stops (for the most part, anyway) in firefights of battle, the helicopter rescue efforts arrive to our medical center within minutes. In addition to getting shot at regularly, the heat, survival, protective gear, and logistical challenges are tremendous. The combat medics endure this daily and are physically and mentally fit, sharp, and experienced. The medics (essentially paramedics with flight environment and survival training) provide ACLS/ATLS, fluids and resuscitation like any medical response in the US, only within the fog of combat operations.

L. Folio (ed.), *Combat Radiology: Diagnostic Imaging of Blast and Ballistic Injuries*,
DOI 10.1007/978-1-4419-5854-9_5, © Springer Science+Business Media, LLC 2010

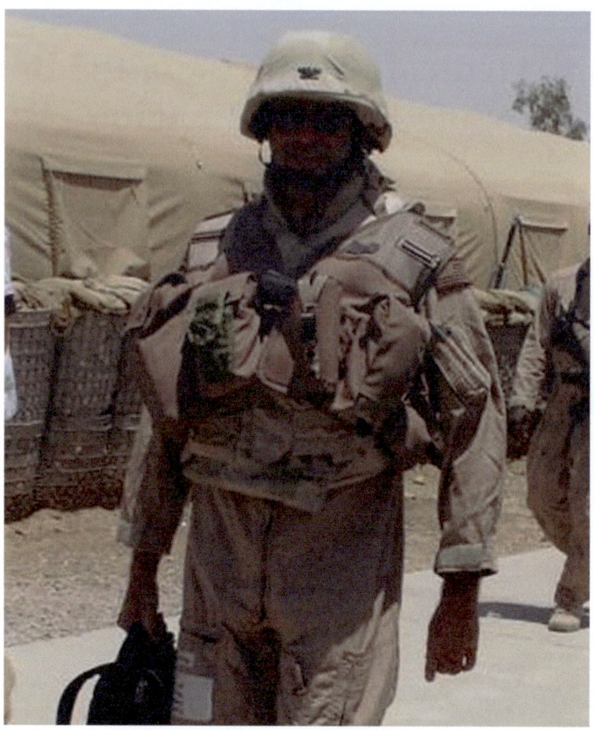

Fig. 5.1 Photo of my preparing to transport a severely injured casualty from one combat hospital in Iraq to another. Radiologists with other medical specialties such as aerospace medicine may be called upon to transport patients on medical evacuation missions

As a flight surgeon, I can only empathize with the conditions that these true heros endure regularly. See Fig. 5.1 for a photo of me preparing to transport a casualty from one combat hospital to another for follow-up care. Note the survival vest to include weapon with rounds on top of the heavy body armor (Fig. 5.2).

5.2   Imaging Advances in Deployed Combat Hospitals

One of the first imaging advances a casualty experiences in Air Force Theater Hospitals is the ultrasound. After the trauma CBAs and continued urgent life support measures, comes the E-FAST (Extended Focused Abdominal Sonography in Trauma). In addition to the four abdominal quadrant FAST for abdominal fluid (e.g., Morrison's pouch), pleural and pericardial fluid surveillance, a look for pneumothorax is obtained for instant information on these important parameters. This policy is AOR wide among all echelons for standardized care. Radiologists can play various roles in the E-FAST, however, are performed mostly by the ED docs and trauma surgeons.

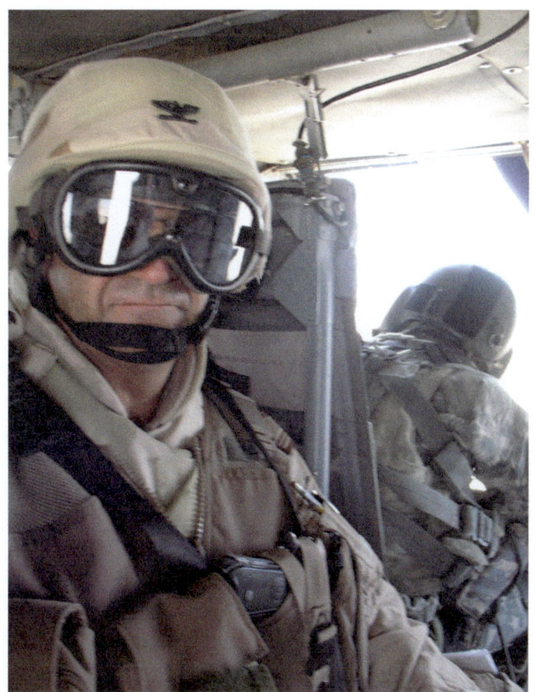

Fig. 5.2 Photo taken within a UH-60 Blackhawk helicopter capable of transporting six litter patients at a time. Note again the survival gear to include M9 weapon all doctors are issued

Ultrasound is also commonly used in the ICU and wards for guided fluid drainage (for fluid collections in the chest, empyemas, abscesses, etc.) not significantly different than many medical centers. Since there is no role for MR in combat as of this writing, MSK US can be of tremendous value. Lastly, research is underway at USU to evaluate and train physicians to use US guidance for foreign body retrieval in blast casualties.

Although fixed fluoroscopy is not commonplace in deployed settings, direct digital C-Arms in the operating rooms have helped vascular/orthopedic surgeons and interventional radiologists perform procedures that rival many university medical centers and trauma hospitals. See Fig. 5.3, for example, C-Arm image capture of a coil placement into a pseudoaneurysm created by a GSW to the neck. See also Figs. 5.4–5.7 for CTA and coiling and postcoiling of pseudoaneurysm. More information on this casualty saved by our resourceful team of providers can be found in Military Medicine [1].

5.3 Anatomic Positioning System and Trajectory Analysis

Imaging advances on the battlefield include recent experience with MDCT and rapid MPR, and 3D volume rendered images to accurately guide trauma surgeons to involved regions and organs more effectively. For example, with CTA and MPR, a radiologist can quickly determine the wound path of a projectile (blast fragment or

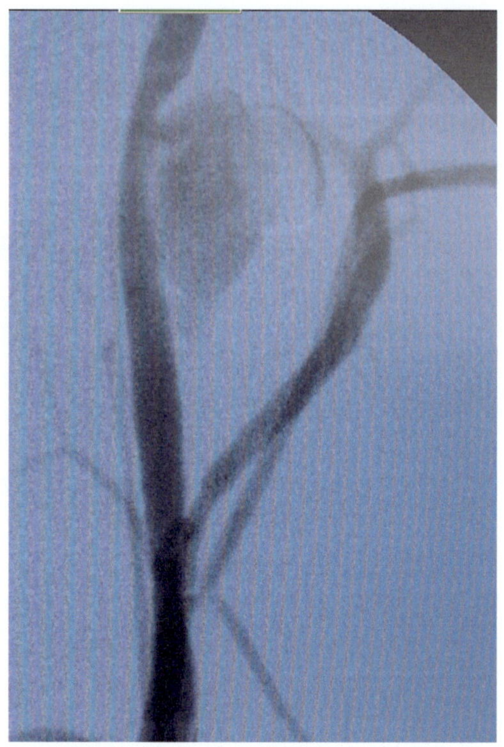

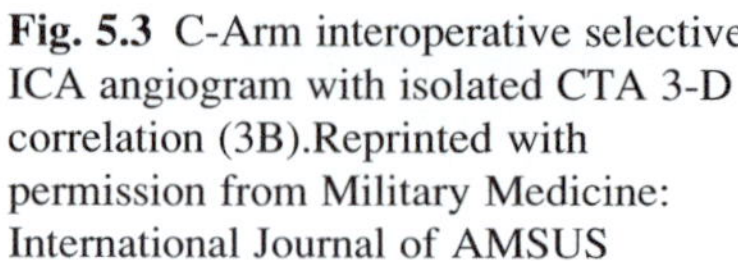

Fig. 5.3 C-Arm interoperative selective ICA angiogram with isolated CTA 3-D correlation (3B).Reprinted with permission from Military Medicine: International Journal of AMSUS

GSW) and demonstrate to the ED doc and/or surgeon the path and potential organ, major vessel involvement [2]. Backus and Folio described these reconstructed MPR's that were off-axis from the cardinal planes as complex planes to include para-axial, para-sagittal, and para-coronal, depending on the closest parent cardinal plane (axial, sagittal, coronal) for consistent reporting and epidemiology.

Beyond the immediate patient care benefits or accurately assessing organ damage, extrapolation of the wound path to a trajectory outside the body can help investigators at the scene determine the location of a sniper based on extrapolated angles, for example. Knowing distance, body orientation or height of sniper, investigators can use the information from the trauma experienced radiologist to determine unknowns. Trajectory analysis has helped identify sniper locations, differentiate from terrorist from friendly fire, and helped catch sniper teams in warfare to help prevent this deadly activity.

The other relatively new concept includes APS or Anatomical Positioning System for accurately and consistently describing retained blast and ballistic fragment locations in a standard fashion. We are currently studying this concept along with the trajectory analysis to evaluate intra-observer accuracy with known fragment locations. We hope to determine trajectory angles to within 5° of azimuth and altitude and fragment location to within a centimeter from a single reference

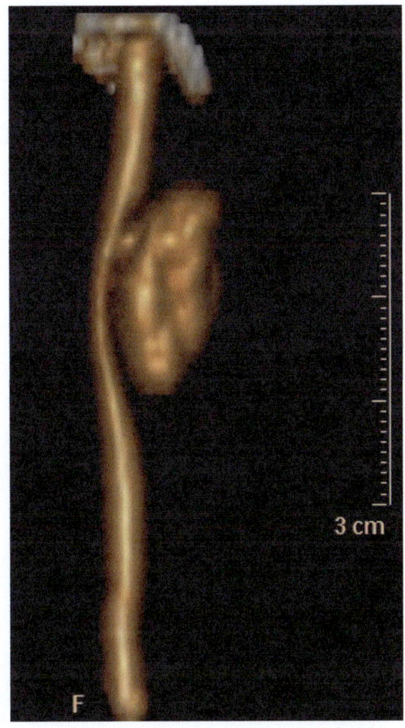

Fig. 5.4 Isolated three-dimensional reformatted image of CT Angiogram showing the internal carotid pseudoaneurysm that correlates well with C-arm angiogram. Reprinted with permission from Military Medicine: International Journal of AMSUS

point. We are also looking into developing an overall fragment score based on size, number, and distribution of fragments for wounded warriors for long-term follow-up on them as individuals and for standard comparison with morbidity and mortality. Long-term research on war wounds, many in the complex planes described, may be easier to track if the terminology is consistent. In addition, for those individuals exposed to two, three, or even more blast injuries (not uncommon in war), retained fragments from past injuries can be differentiated from new blast fragments. In addition, identifying the migration of retained fragments will be enhanced by consistent tracking and documenting as projectiles migrate through vessels in the body.

Determining trajectory angles using standard terminology in complex planes and quantifiable angles can be consistently described with complex planes. The classic anatomic planes are shown in Fig. 5.8. Each of the classic planes is 90° offset from two other planes, similar to the cardinal directions of a compass. Cardinal navigational points include north, south, east, and west on a compass. Intermediate planes are introduced here as variations from the classic planes (see Fig. 5.9). Any plane from pure axial to 45° offset from axial is described here as para-axial. Then from that midway point between axial and the other two planes, a description of para-sagittal or para-coronal are appropriate. It should be kept in mind that all planar rotation refers to an infinite number of planes.

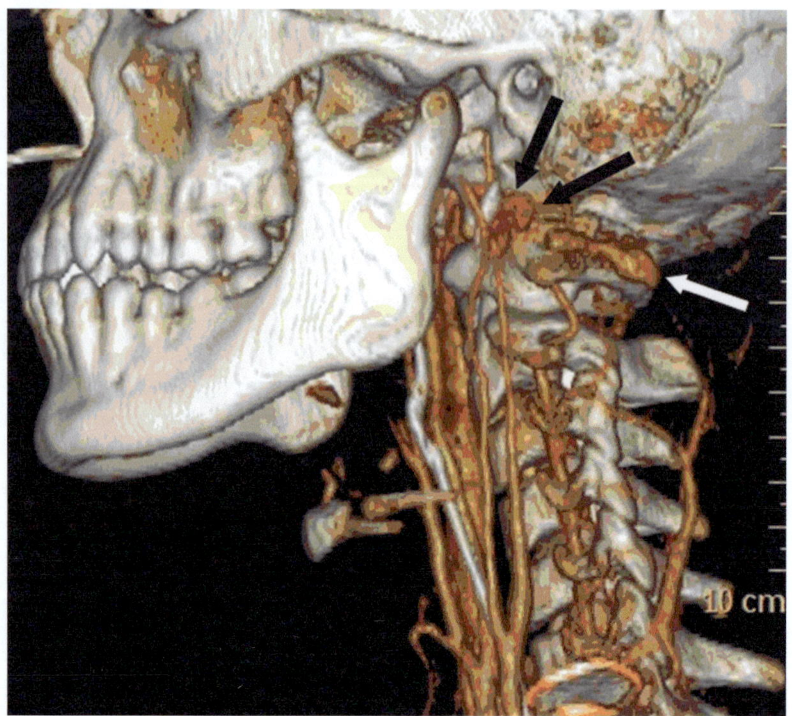

Fig. 5.5 Three-dimensional reformatted image of CT Angiogram showing the internal carotid pseudoaneurysm (*black arrows*) and small vertebral pseudoaneurysm (*white arrow*). Reprinted with permission from Military Medicine: International Journal of AMSUS

An important element to understand complex planes requires an understanding of anatomic axes [3]. Pilots have defined and named rotation around each of the three axes of their aircraft in order to clarify communication as seen in Fig. 5.10. Pivoting around the X-axis is "roll," around the Y-axis is "pitch," and around the Z-axis is "yaw." Pilots use degrees to describe how much they have pivoted around the appropriate axis, such as "Pitch up 10° to climb." That direction is easily translated to rotate 10° around the Y-axis. It is concise, clear, and easy to convert and describe.

See Fig. 5.11 to show how anatomic axes relate to established axes in aviation. Degree deviations from the classic planes could be used similarly to precisely describe complex planes intermediate between the classic planes of section (Fig. 5.12). When referring to CT however, the x- and y-axes are switched to accommodate for pixel locations on image space. This has recently been applied to tumor navigation and identification [4].

The following is an example how to qualitatively describe these starting with the *para-sagittal plane*. In this example, the difference is between a para-sagittal plane and the classic sagittal plane. See Fig. 5.13 showing an example para-sagittal plane.

Fig. 5.6 Selective coiling of
pseudoaneurysm performed by our
deployed interventional radiologist and
vascular surgeon in an isoshelter
operating room in the tent facility.
Reprinted with permission from Military
Medicine: International Journal
of AMSUS

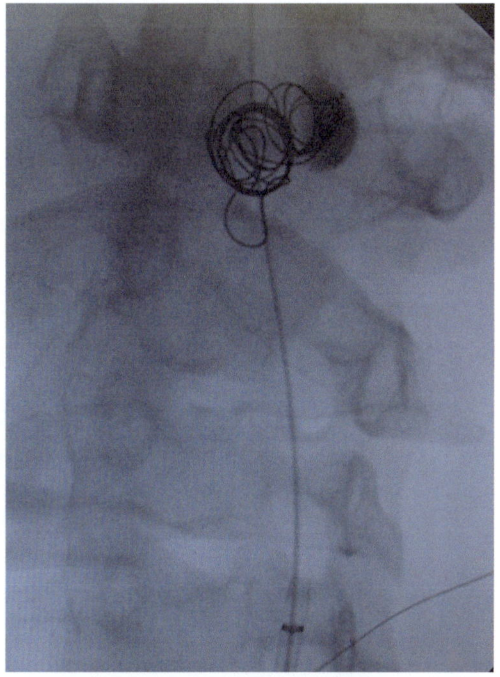

The para-sagittal plane drawn in this example is rotated around the anatomic Z-axis 25° left. One can describe any para-sagittal plane intermediate between the sagittal and coronal plane by defining the rotation around the Z-axis relative to the "pure" sagittal. These planes would all be between 0 and 45° (for purposes of description) total arc. A para-sagittal plane intermediate between sagittal and coronal could be described by yaw left or right (from the patient's viewpoint). For example, a radiologist could specify a para-sagittal plane yawed (or rotated around the Z-axis) 30° right. Once past the 45° point, I call this the para-coronal plane.

A *para-axial plane* is intermediate between the axial and coronal plane by defining the pitch up or pitch down from "pure" axial. These planes would all be between up/down 45° or a 90° (for purposes of description) total arc. Para-axial planes intermediate between axial and sagittal can be described by their roll (or rotation around the X-axis). For example, a radiologist could specify a para-axial plane rolled (or rotated around the X-axis) 30° right.

A *para-coronal plane* intermediate between coronal and sagittal could be described by the yaw (or rotation around the Z-axis) while a para-coronal plane intermediate between coronal and axial could be described by pitch (or rotation around the Y-axis) forward or backward. The intersection of two skewed (off-axis) planes results in a line that represents the trajectory of the missile, inside and outside of the body.

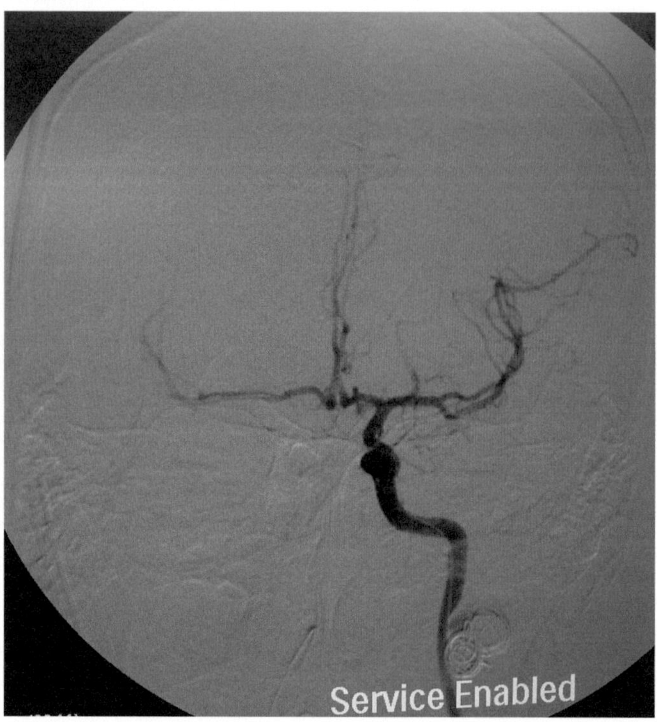

Fig. 5.7 Selective ICA showing adequate intracerebral patency. Note the coils inhibiting flow into pseudoaneurysm. Reprinted with permission from Military Medicine: International Journal of AMSUS

5.4   Compass Analogy

The classic planes are not unlike the cardinal directions on a compass (Fig. 5.14a) or the geometric x, y, z coordinate system. The degree headings of a compass (Fig. 5.14b) will relate to the anatomic quantifiable trajectories. Using this same analogy, intermediate or complex planes introduced here are like intermediate headings on a compass such as NW (NorthWest, or the midpoint between North and West). The direction between North and NorthWest can be further defined as NNW (North-NorthWest). Similarly, a plane intermediate between axial and coronal, but closer to axial could be described as axial-axialcoronal (AAC) (Fig. 5.15). This can also be true about each of the anatomic axes, see Fig. 5.16 for an example.

Taking that one step further, one could apply the radial degrees around each of several axes like the degrees on a compass (Fig. 5.17) to precisely describe intermediate planes, but a more intuitive system using fewer than 360° can be devised.

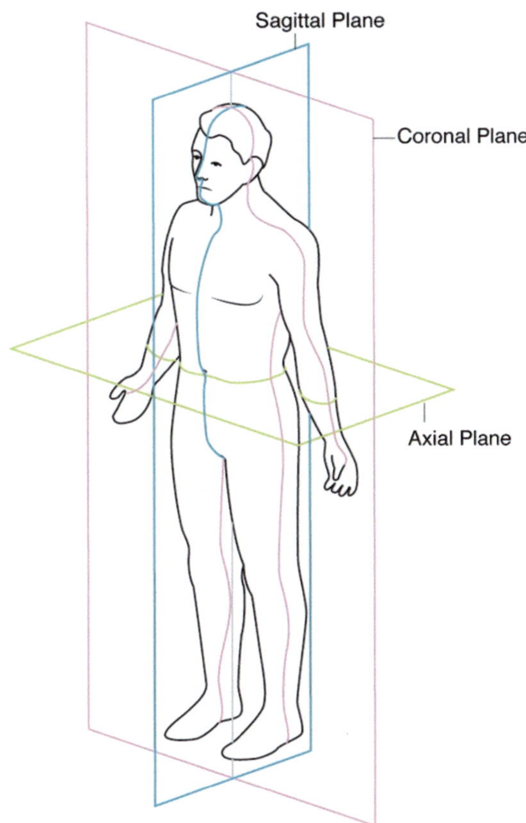

Fig. 5.8 The basic anatomic planes, axial, coronal, and sagittal. Drawing by Sofia Echelmeyer

5.5 Construction of the Trajectory Plane(s) from the CT Dataset

Radiologists typically interpret CT datasets by scrolling through axial CT scan slices on a daily basis. With the introduction of MDCT in recent years, it has become more common to complement the traditional interpretive process with a more complex viewing of volumetrically acquired datasets [5]. Trajectories have been analyzed in the past, both by administration of contrast and by CT [6]. Recent work from Walter Reed Medical Center has demonstrated identification of trajectories using Anatomic Positioning System Cartesian coordinates and image space/table position on CT [7]. This was further validated on analysis of combat casualty data from Iraq where investigators were able to identify wound paths consistently and qualitatively described them in 90% of trajectories. We further demonstrated that radiologist's measurements using image space and table position were able to

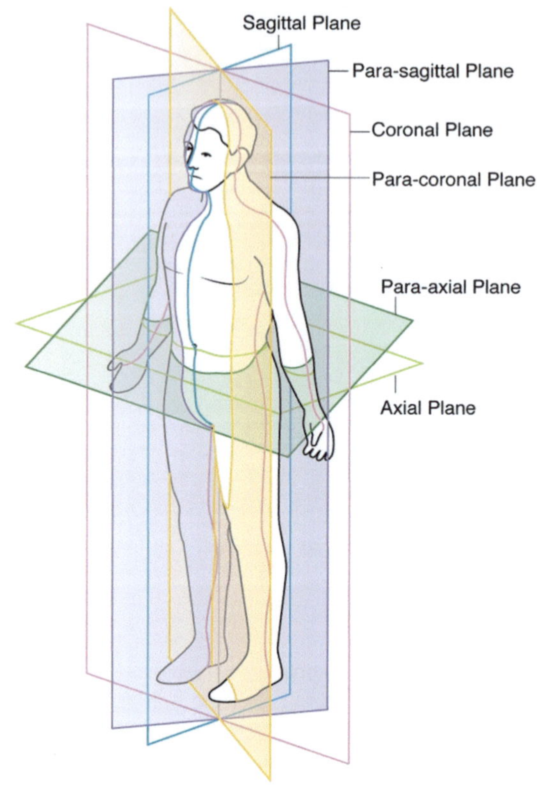

Fig. 5.9 Artist's representation of complex planes is now possible with modern imaging. The complex planes and nomenclature are defined here as intermediaries of the simple planes described above. Each of the planes here are 30° off their parent planes as an example. Reprinted with permission from Military Medicine: International Journal of AMSUS

be mapped consistently enough to calculate the qualitative descriptions of trajectories at the same rate [8]. We created a Cartesian coordinate calculator that could also calculate qualitative trajectories from radiologist measurements using Excel.

Basically this means that radiologists can tilt the plane on any level which is called Multi-Planar Reformation (MPR) [9]. This capability is especially helpful in determining trajectories of blast and ballistic fragments, or resultant pathways when able. This further assists trauma radiologists in providing detailed descriptions to trauma surgeons on an immediate basis as to what anatomical structures are potentially involved, or not involved. This is key in radiologic diagnosis, triage of multiple casualties say from a blast, and guiding trauma surgeons to operating with greater precision. An example of an application of this methodology is described here using a case of a GSW to the chest. Additional cases are reviewed to show how this can apply to other types of projectiles in various anatomic regions.

The first case is a 31-year-old active duty male deployed troop that suffered a gunshot wound (GSW) to the left chest. More detail about the clinical information is available in the author's prior work in Military Medicine [10]. This combat casualty was immediately medevaced from field conditions to a combat hospital in Iraq. The patient was hemodynamically stable in the ER, with the following AP

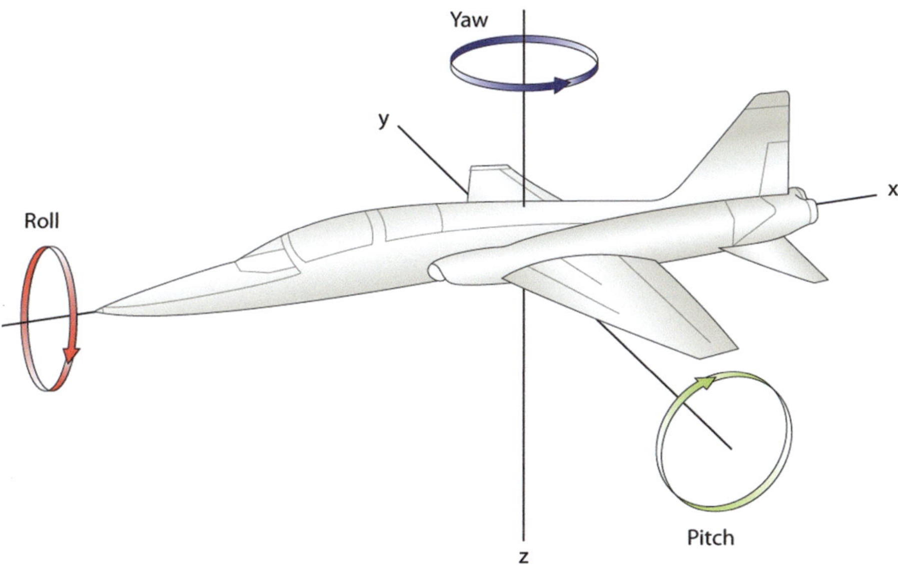

Fig. 5.10 In the aviation sciences, axes are assigned to each possible movement of aircraft for descriptive purposes. Reprinted with permission from Military Medicine: International Journal of AMSUS

chest image obtained to evaluate involvement and rough missile trajectory estimate. This, combined with the clinical observation of single entrance wound to upper left chest anteriorly, demonstrated the bullet overlying the mediastinum, likely posterior. Figure 5.17 demonstrates the bullet overlying the mediastinum, likely posterior, based on isolated anterior entrance noted clinically. Figure 5.18 is reformatted para-axial slice showing the obvious pathway of the missile. The longitudinal homogenous pathway from anterior to posterior aligns with the bullet and entrance. This is the permanent cavity left from the missile. Figure 5.19 shows the parasagittal plane along the tilted trajectory and can serve as a scout for the para-axial plane determined by pivoting around the known path points.

The first step in trajectory analysis is for the radiologist to walk to the Emergency Department (ED), trauma unit, or less optimally CT and see the patient and wound locations. Ideally, face to face interaction with the ED physician and trauma surgeon will optimize the scan protocol based on the injuries, help determine the wound path, and optimally guide the trauma surgeons based on involved vasculature and organ damage. Based on the most expeditious protocols for that casualty, image acquisition is next. Institution CT protocols often include volumetric data acquisition. Volumetric acquisition is ideal to recreate the data in any plane about any axis. Then postprocessing or image dataset manipulation is done at a diagnostic radiologist workstation or networked PC with dedicated DICOM software. At that point, one identifies the classic plane that the complex plane (described earlier) most closely resembles. However, more precision is available by defining the deviation from the classic plane using the terminology already established in aviation.

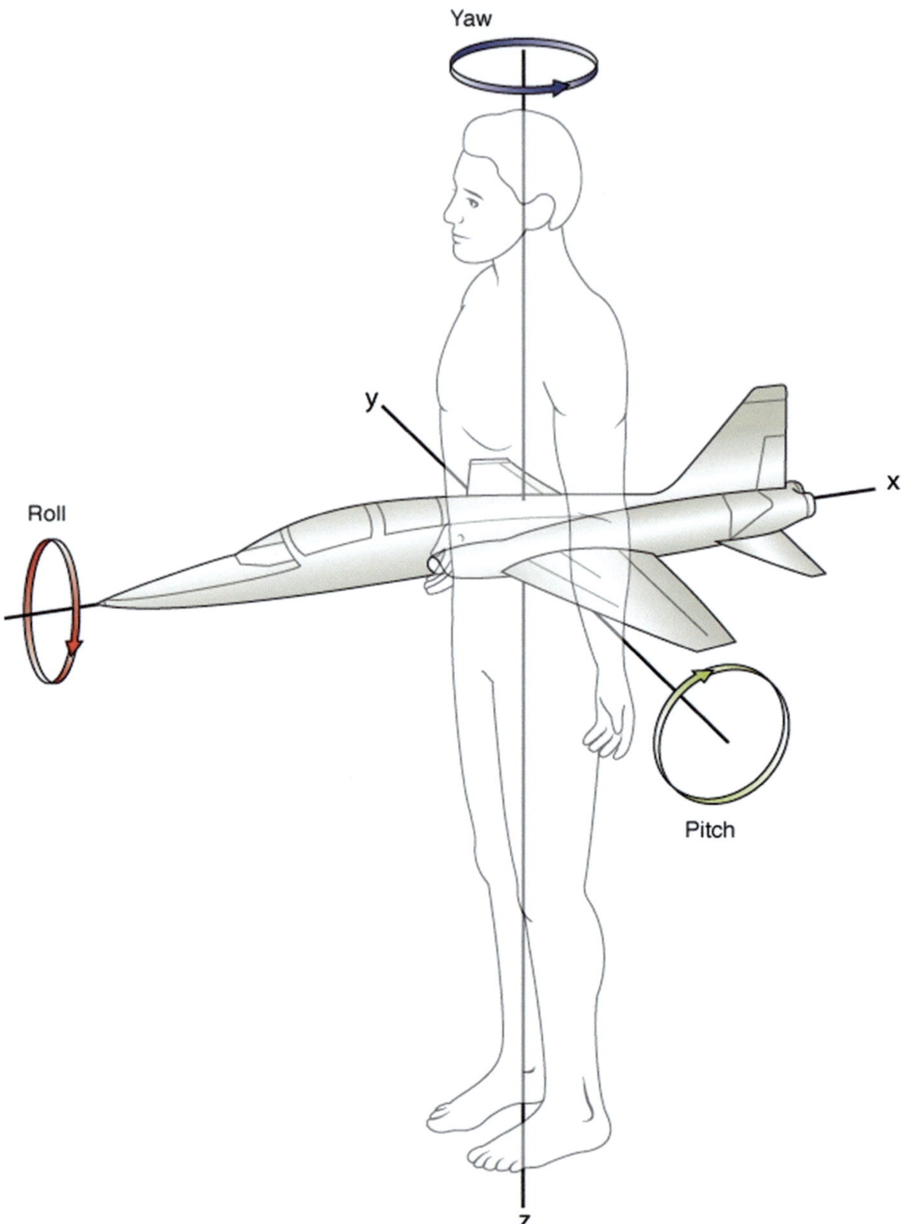

Fig. 5.11 In aerospace medicine, axes are applied to the human body as a pilot is seated in an aircraft, to parallel aviation sciences nomenclature. Reprinted with permission from Military Medicine: International Journal of AMSUS

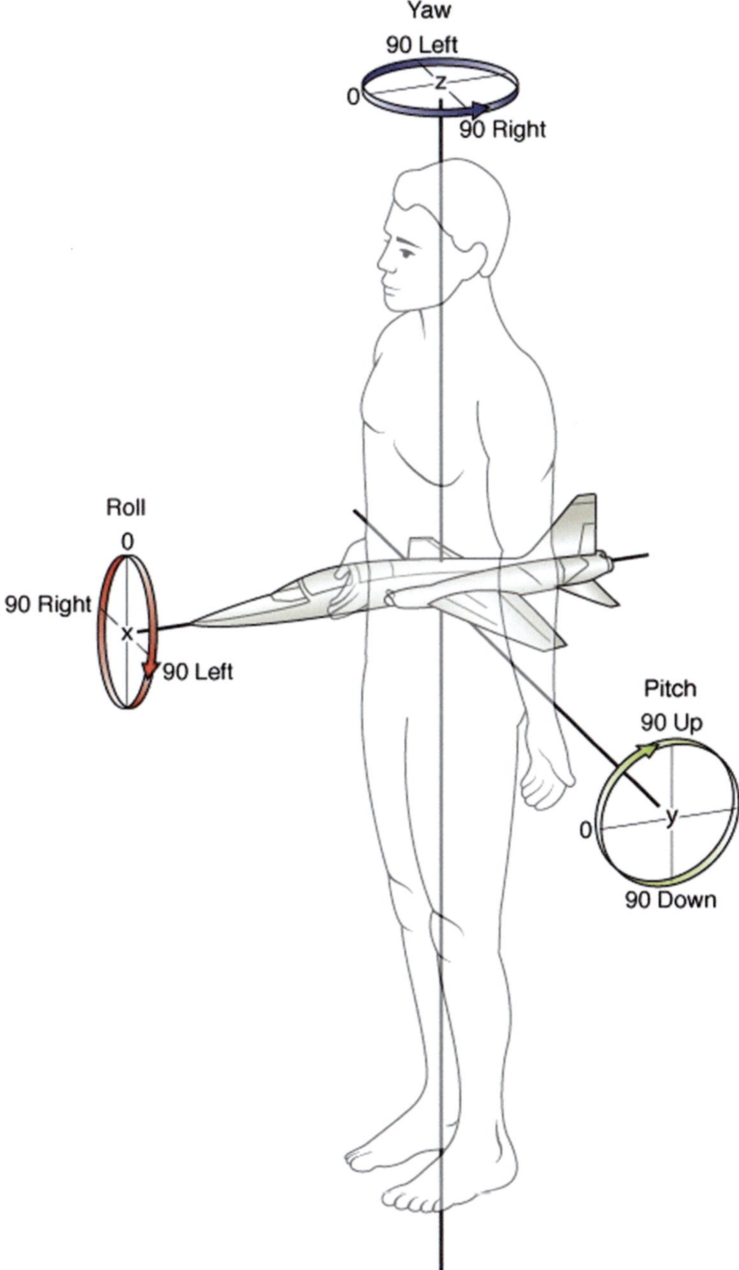

Fig. 5.12 Taking the descriptions a step further, degrees of planes relative to axes can be applied in all directions, about all axes. Reprinted with permission from Military Medicine: International Journal of AMSUS

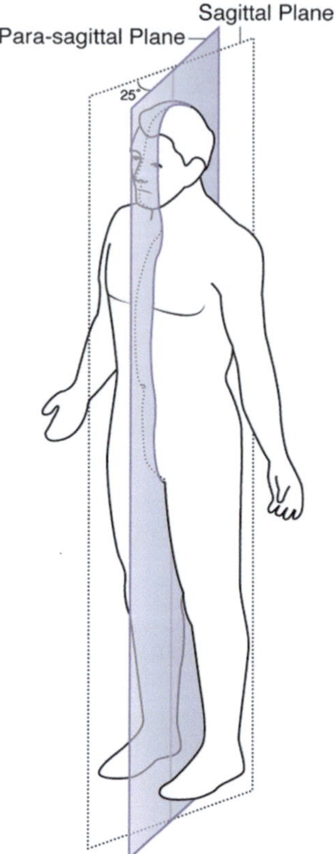

Fig. 5.13 This drawing shows a para-sagittal plane of 25° pivoted about the anatomic Z-axis toward the left. Reprinted with permission from Military Medicine: International Journal of AMSUS

5.6 The Trajectory Mapping Is Accomplished in the Following Manner

When a radiologist gets to a validated path point such as ballistic fragment, entrance, exit, or fracture, the plane is pivoted about that point, in attempt to find other positive pathway identifiers. The case analyzed should have a simple path that is traceable. Many perforating injuries seen in combat from high-velocity weapons fit this criteria as they do not expend their energy in the body. Even paths that ricochet can often be analyzed. Many low-velocity injuries are more chaotic as they expend their energy within the body tissues and may not be traceable. Para-sagittal and/or para-coronal reference slices or "scouts" are often useful for showing the relative planar angles. See Fig. 5.19 once again for our first example para-sagittal of lowest axial plane (1), the most superior axial plane (2) at entrance wound (seen on another slice), and resultant para-axial plane (3) that was ultimately found by this process. This initial case highlights quantification of degrees around axis (Figs. 5.20 and 5.21). Basically, the entrance and exit are found on axial, the middle slice is determined, then the axial slice is tilted by MPR while using the sagittal (or coronal) view as a reference. This can be done from any combination of the three basic

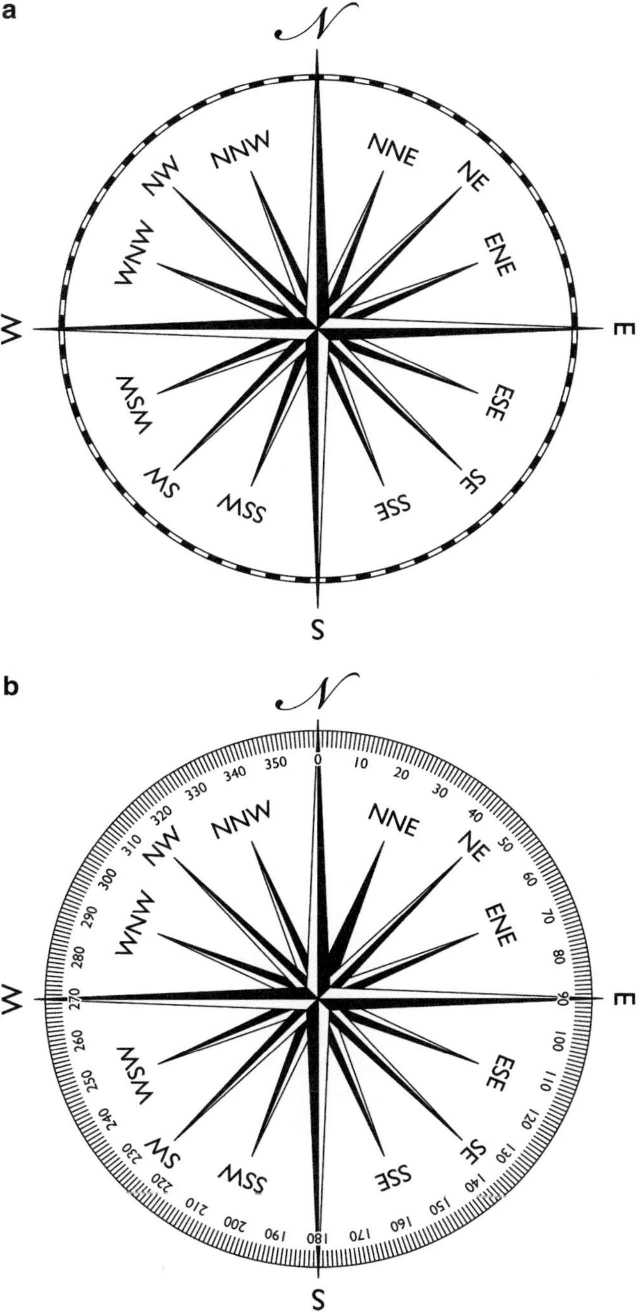

Fig. 5.14 (**a**) Cardinal headings of a compass rose. Drawing by Sofia Echelmeyer. Reprinted with permission from Military Medicine: International Journal of AMSUS. (**b**) Degree headings of a compass rose. Drawing by Sofia Echelmeyer. Reprinted with permission from Military Medicine: International Journal of AMSUS

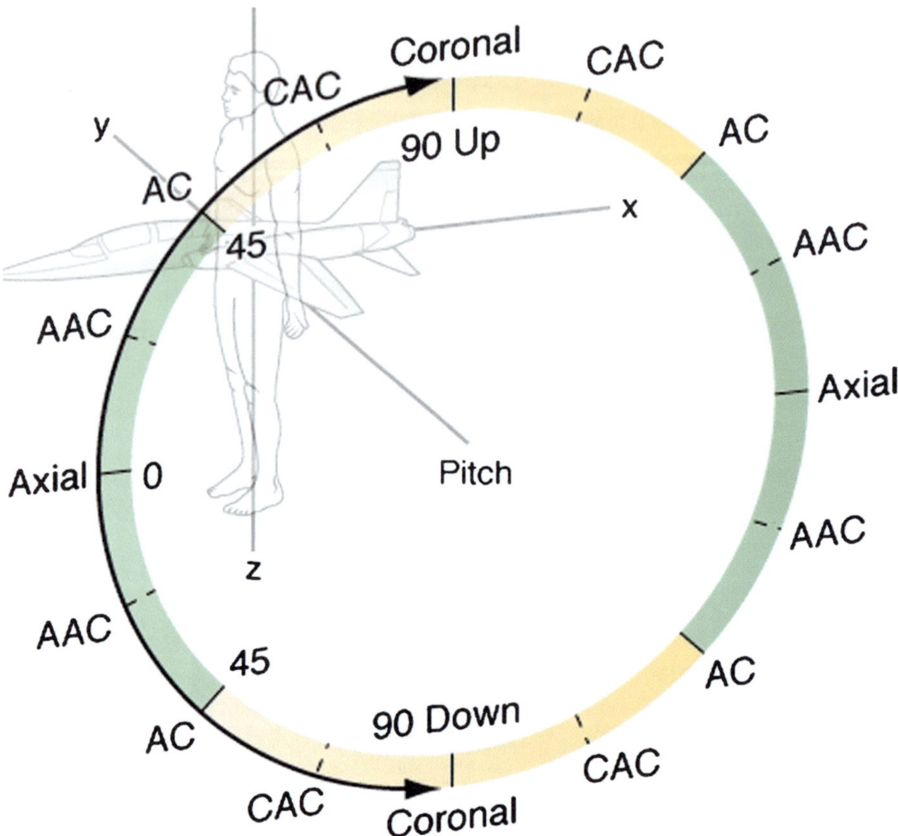

Fig. 5.15 Superimposing the anatomic *y*-axis with the aircraft example allows one to see how pitch can be described in a number of segmented, defined complex intermediary planes similar to how a compass can be further divided into NW and NWW. Drawing by Sofia Echelmeyer. Reprinted with permission from Military Medicine: International Journal of AMSUS

anatomic planes as a starting point. In addition to skin wounds as clues to missile path, fractured bones, remaining metal fragments, subcutaneous air can help determine path. Figure 5.22 shows the para-axial orientation in the body for descriptive purposes, and Fig. 5.23 to demonstrate quantification on one axis. These figures are reprinted from Folio et al [11].

The second plane can be seen by referring back to Fig. 5.13 as a para-sagittal plane yawed 25° left. A three-dimensional wound path (such as the path of a projectile or fragment) can be described by the intersection of two two-dimensional complex planes (see Fig. 5.24). The bullet path is described by the line of intersection between para-axial pitched up 14° and para-sagittal yawed 25° left. Figure 5.25 is a collage of the two complex planes along the bullet path, demonstrating the upward and rightward angle of the path in another graphic form. Many of the bullet paths currently seen in Iraq are caused by snipers shooting from a high position,

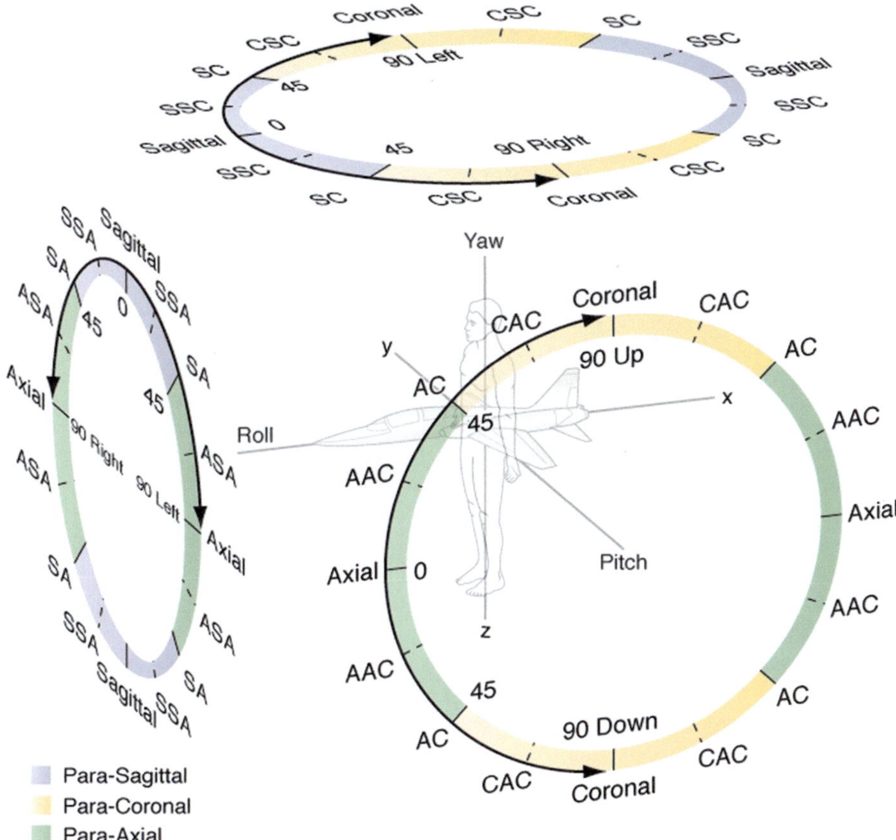

Fig. 5.16 This drawing shows how intermediary planes can be described about all axes. Reprinted with permission from Military Medicine: International Journal of AMSUS

such as atop a building or through a window. This can be seen by the extended bullet path in Fig. 5.26, where the first plane is a para-axial pitched up 14°.

5.7 Additional Cases Presented to Highlight Complex Plane Application

The following are some other examples of penetrating blast or ballistic trauma to highlight trajectory analysis and complex plane description. The next case is another penetrating lung injury, less severe than the first one presented. This is another example of superior to inferior trajectory, likely a sniper, with less bleeding than the first case. Figure 5.27 shows the permanent cavity with air as opposed to blood in the other case. The surrounding consolidative opacities represent contusion

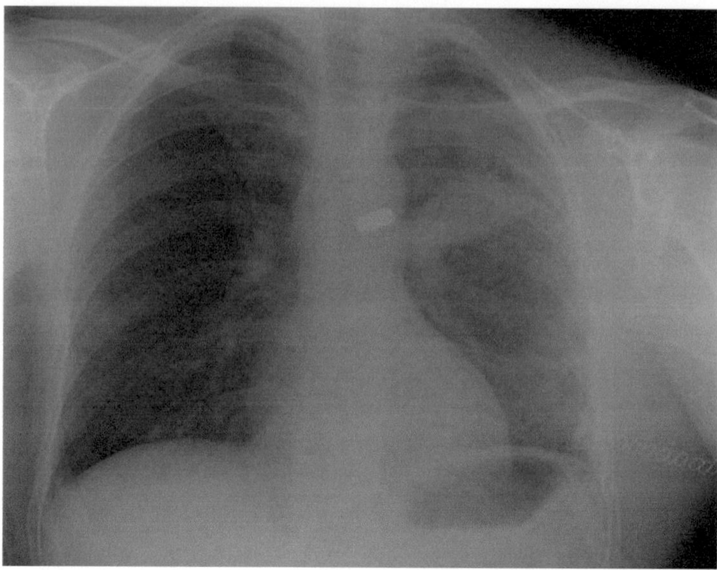

Fig. 5.17 GSW chest X-ray. Reprinted with permission from Military Medicine: International Journal of AMSUS

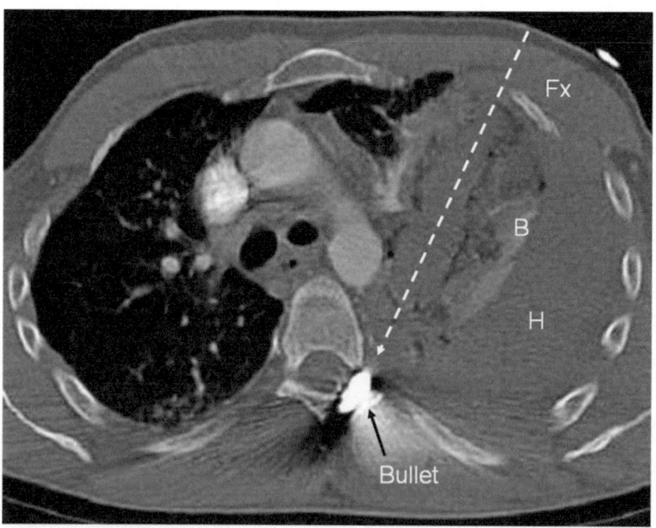

Fig. 5.18 Para-axial CT showing wound path. Reprinted with permission from Military Medicine: International Journal of AMSUS

Fig. 5.19 Para-sagittal MPR showing downward angle from sniper shot. Reprinted with permission from Military Medicine: International Journal of AMSUS

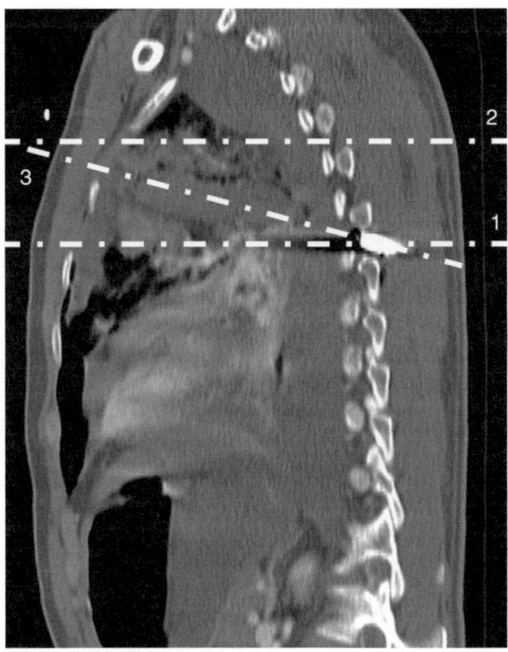

Fig. 5.20 The same para-sagittal MPR showing trajectory at 14° pitch down. Reprinted with permission from Military Medicine: International Journal of AMSUS

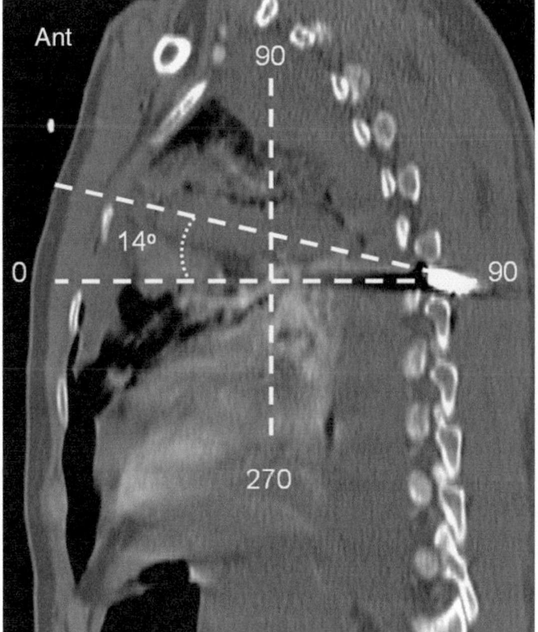

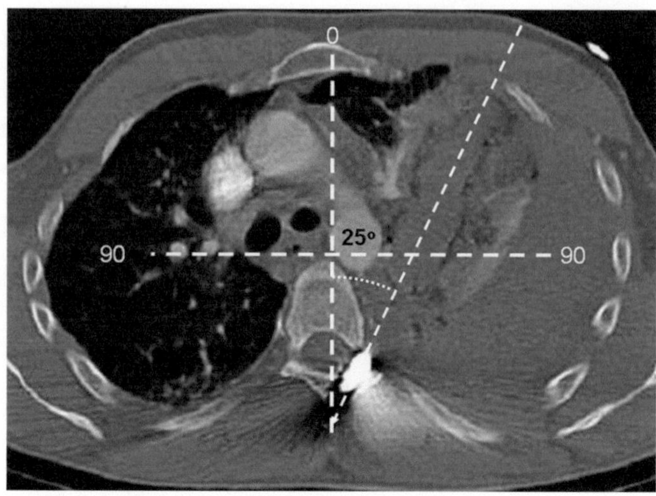

Fig. 5.21 The para-axial MPR showing trajectory 25° toward the patients left. Reprinted with permission from Military Medicine: International Journal of AMSUS

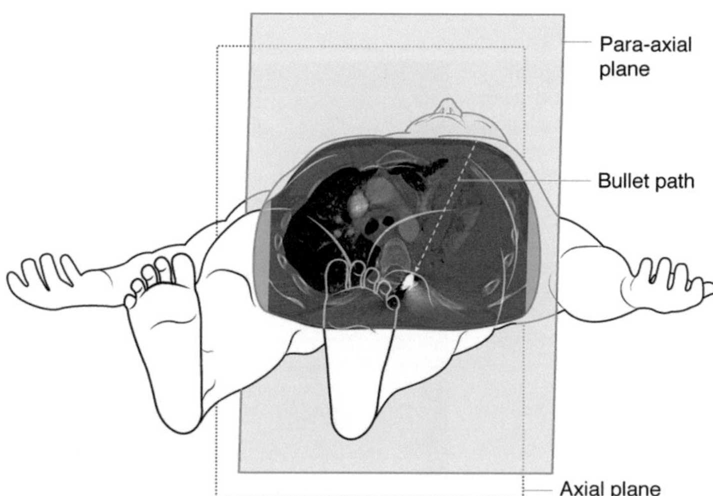

Fig. 5.22 This drawing shows how the para-axial CT is oriented in the body. Reprinted with permission from Military Medicine: International Journal of AMSUS

from the tumbling of the bullet approximating the temporary cavity. The trajectory appears to go through the intact scapula, this is due to a different position of the scapula during the injury. This gunshot was from anterior to posterior, entering the patient's left infraclavicular region, exiting further to the patient's left posterior

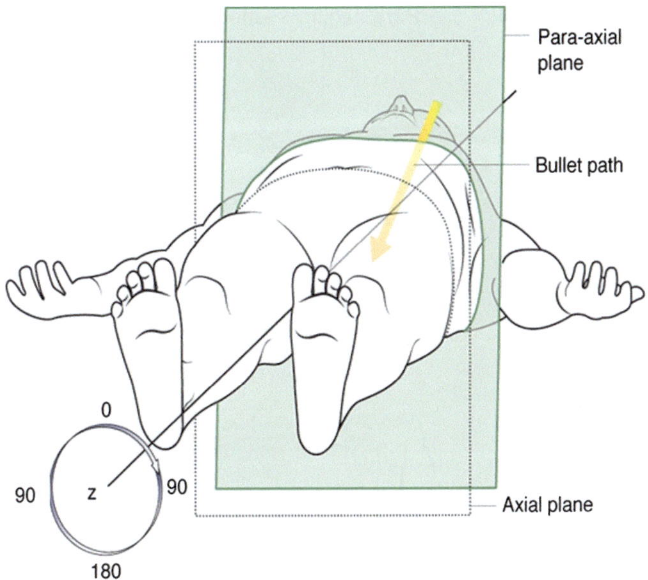

Fig. 5.23 This drawing shows the orientation of the para-axial slice, the para-sagittal rotation of the GSW trajectory. Reprinted with permission from Military Medicine: International Journal of AMSUS

chest. Figure 5.28 shows the quantitative para-sagittal orientation on the para-axial CT MPR.

The next case is of a casualty suffering a grenade injury to the face and neck that has been well described [12]. Figure 5.29 demonstrates the para-axial plane that lines up the fragment entrance and resting place near right lateral ventricle. On closer inspection and planar reformation, the para-sagittal trajectory plane was further determined, eventually enabling accurate incident analysis. See Figs. 5.30 and 5.31 for artists' rendition demonstrating how trajectory detection allowed me to discover damage to the carotid siphon, the tilt of the head during the blast, and the location of the grenade when it detonated. This case highlights how parallel para-axial interpretation based on reference fragments helps find other missiles and associated vascular damage.

A case illustrating a simple but definite path is seen on para-axial images of the liver of a child in close proximity to a blast that has also been well described [13]. Note the large irregular fragment in the right upper abdomen in Fig. 5.32. The projectile traveled anterior to posterior, from right to left. The right elbow was part of the trajectory path evident on the CT scout (Fig. 5.33 shows them both on the same trajectory plane) by severely comminuted fracture and metal fragments. This is further delineated on CT (Figs. 5.34 and 5.35). The right anterior rib at this level is fractured, indicating inclusion in path making this easier to map the missile path. Note the right arm also demonstrates some metallic remnants. The right arm was

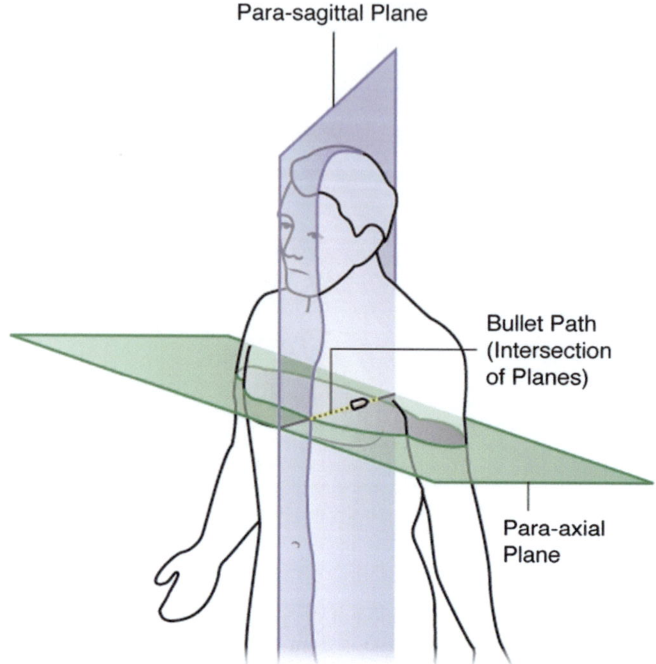

Fig. 5.24 The two complex planes intersecting to create the line representing the trajectory. Reprinted with permission from Military Medicine: International Journal of AMSUS

closer to the body and more anterior at the time of the blast. The determination of arm position can also be helpful in incident analysis with multiple victims from a firefight.

When it comes to recreating the scene or determining multiple missiles' paths in individual victims, another useful determinate that is well described is the keyhole fracture in the skull [14]. See Figs. 5.36 and 5.37 for example, trajectory determination based on orientation of the keyhole that is well described by Jackson. Figures 5.38–5.41 show forces and vectors of initial bullet and resultant bone fragments (which then become the "missile"). Velocity of projectiles is as much of a factor in certain injuries as size [15]. Types of rifles, bores, and bullets are also important factors in wound ballistics [16–18].

One blast victim caught a projectile across his back, perforating the right scapula, traveled through his mid thoracic spine, then through two left ribs evidenced by fractures. Figure 5.42 shows the para-axial reformat showing the entire path on one slice. The projectile then traveled through left arm as well (seen on images not included). The 3D view (Fig. 5.43) shows the path. Scapular involvement (or lack thereof) can sometimes help determine the position of the arms at the time of injury (Figs. 5.44–5.46).

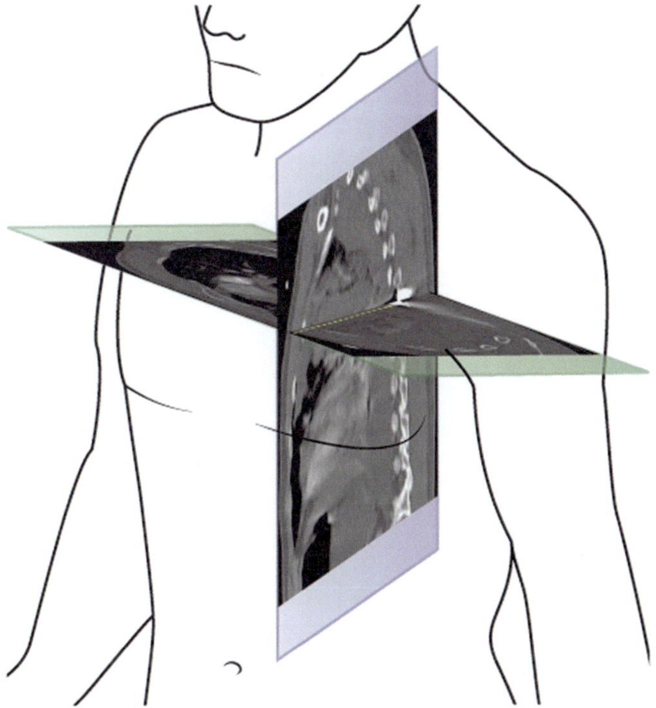

Fig. 5.25 A collage of the two complex plane CT MPRs demonstrating how they intersect at a ray vector describing the trajectory accurately. Reprinted with permission from Military Medicine: International Journal of AMSUS

5.8 Abdominal Trajectories

In the following case, determining the trajectory helped establish associated organ injuries by increasing conspicuity with association along the wound path of a large blast fragment. This case has been well described in the literature [19]. Figures 5.47–5.49 shows an intraperitoneal fragment entered from the back of this child. The para-coronal reformat (Fig. 5.50) demonstrates the path from the left back through the lower pole of the left kidney, through the splenic vasculature (based on a devascularized spleen), the pancreatic tail, diaphragmatic crus then finally residing adjacent to the aorta just superior to the left renal vein. Peritoneal fluid is seen bilaterally; however, there is no evidence of major vascular extravasation. This patient was re-triaged to the operating room at a higher priority level than other patients with less severe injuries (Fig. 5.51).

This next casualty was exposed to a blast from the back and has been described [20]. Figure 5.52 is the scout CT showing the large fragment in the lower abdomen. In Figs. 5.53–5.55para-axial reformats demonstrate a large metal fragment that ended

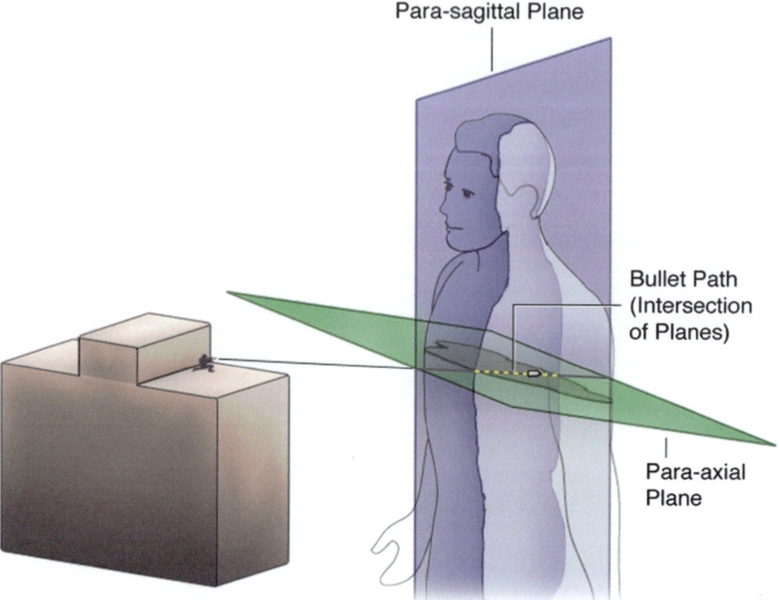

Fig. 5.26 The trajectory extrapolated to the sniper location from a height–distance perspective, and aspect relative to the body at the time of the shot. Reprinted with permission from Military Medicine: International Journal of AMSUS

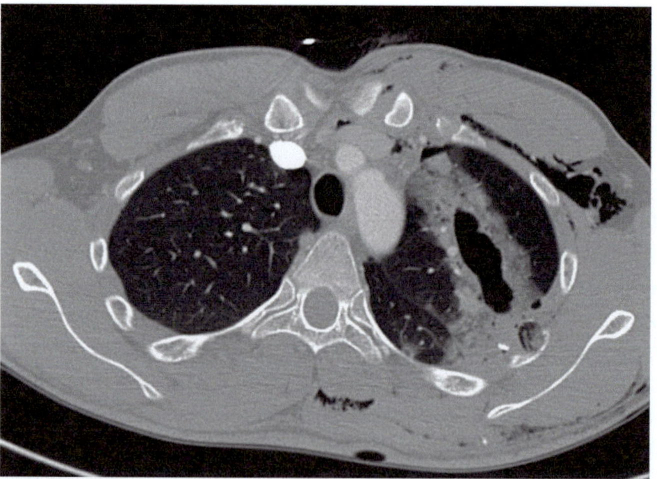

Fig. 5.27 Para-axial CT MPR nicely demonstrating the permanent cavity (linear lucency representing lung laceration) and the temporary cavitation effects of the tumbling bullet

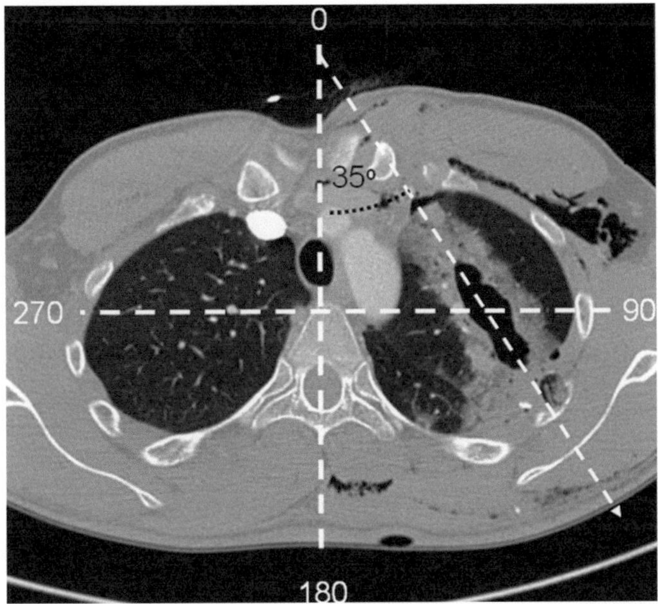

Fig. 5.28 Para-axial CT MPR demonstrating the para-sagittal orientation of the wound path and resultant trajectory

up in the anterior left psoas muscle. The reformats helped demonstrate the lack of intraperitoneal involvement, i.e., this fragment path was shown to be mostly muscular in its trajectory (paravertebral musculature, quadratus lumborum, then psoas). The fractured transverse process, subcutaneous air and soft tissue aberration were all supporting evidence of the missile path. The radiologist in this case worked closely with the ED physician and trauma surgeon to help lower the re-triage status to the operating room since there was likely no bowel perforation or major intra-abdominal process. The operating rooms were full with more critically injured casualties waiting. This again highlights the value of the radiologist presence in the ED and operating rooms with regular interaction of protocolization and preliminary results.

5.9 Ricochet Trajectories

Figure 5.56 highlights a perforating fragment from the back through the right leg that ricocheted superiorly off the right iliac wing that has been well described [21]. Multiplanar reformation in two separate para-axial planes showed that the path was deflected superiorly after striking the iliac wing (Figs. 5.57 and 5.58). This required two reformats: inferior and superior para-axial orientations. This is not uncommon when bone is in the missile path. These reformats helped show that the fragment

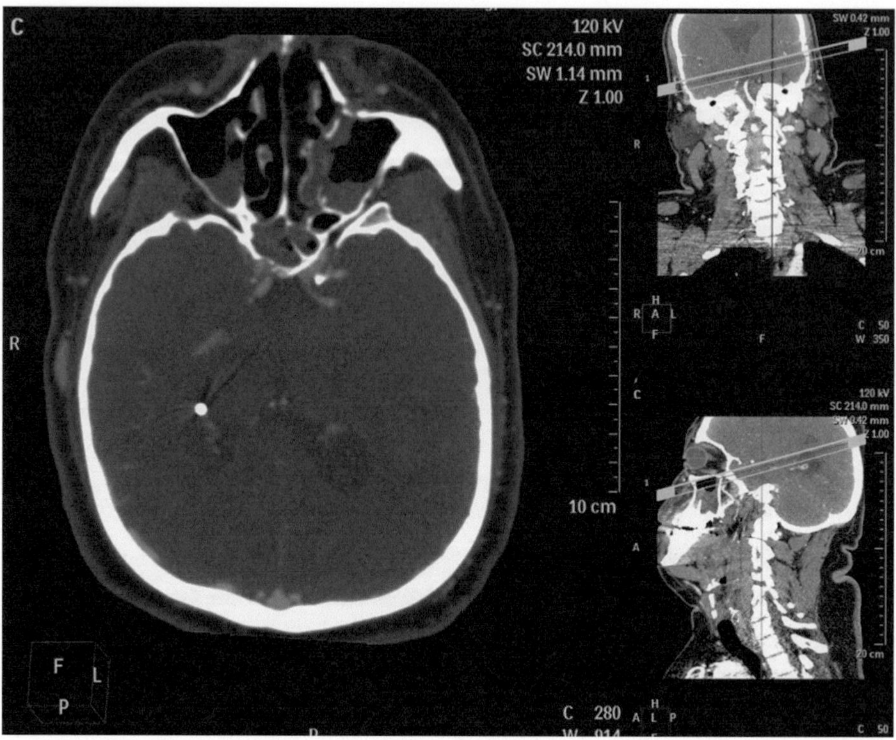

Fig. 5.29 Para-axial CT showing entrance and fragment resting location on one plane. Without lining these up, it would be challenging to determine the damage to the cavernous carotid as we did here

remained extraperitoneal. Although trajectory determination is not as crucial in the abdomen as head, neck, and chest, it can still help identify mystery fragments, or provide clues to potential ureteric, bowel, and/or vessel damage. It should be kept in mind that missiles often ricochet against bone and often change paths as in the previous case. Missiles have also been known to penetrate vasculature and embolize outside the range of entry [22]. For this reason, an even number guide can be applied to demonstrate the need to continue a hunt for an uneven fragment/wound count [23].

Figure 5.59 shows a CXR in a tangential spine injury where ballistic entered through left pectoral muscle anteriorly, between anterior ribs, through lung with a superior to inferior tract, then hit T4 on the left, ricocheted superior exiting also on the left (Figs. 5.60–5.62). This was another sniper shot, missing major vasculature and the spinal canal, and ricocheting superior once again, with fragments further verifying exit from spine through the back. This case has been well described in the literature [24].

Figures 5.63 and 5.64 demonstrate a missile trajectory through the spinal canal at a high level (C4) with slight deflection. Quantitative description of the trajectory to

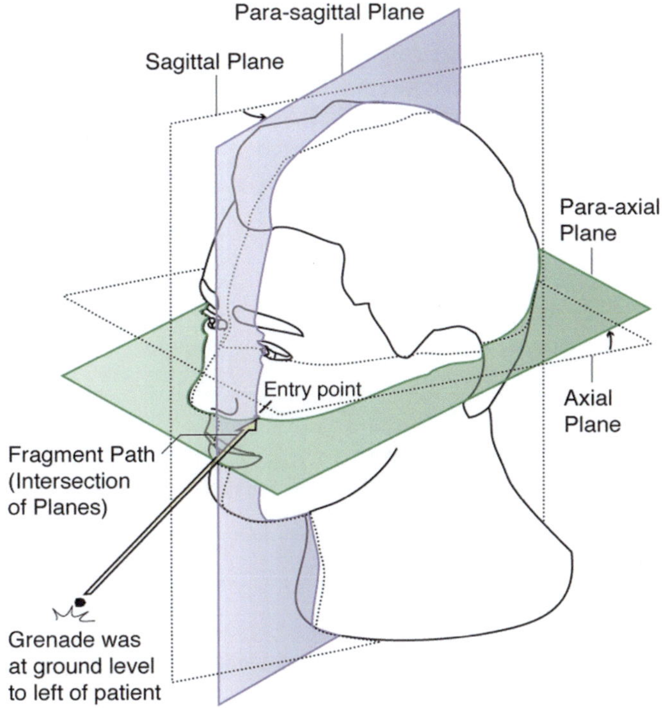

Fig. 5.30 Drawing showing the blast fragment entrance and trajectory to the face that ended up in the left lateral ventricle

include anatomic locations included in the pathway, provide descriptive text for a report or more importantly dynamic triage in combat. For example, some deployed locations in the battlefield have CT capability, however, do not have a radiologist on site. There are often times the CT data cannot be transmitted due to regular power outages, bandwidth limitations, security patches, or business rules. Having the textual report and precise location of trajectory and fragment and anatomic locations could help triage nonsurvivable injuries for urgent helicopter evacuation to higher surgical capabilities. Following trajectory mapping described here, one can appreciate a single ricochet at a slight angle after impacting the left cervical lamina.

To help validate the wound path identification, angle, and resultant trajectory determination, initial research on phantoms and anatomic ballistic simulators by Folio and Fischer et al is demonstrating consistent determinations of known sniper trajectories [25]. Ballistic testing of synthetic legs (donated by Operative Experiences, Inc. out of Kennedyville, MD) originally designed for teaching surgery is showing excellent correlation of angles shot by a .30-06 rifle (similar muzzle velocity as weapons used by terrorists). See Fig. 5.65 for sniper bench/clinometer,

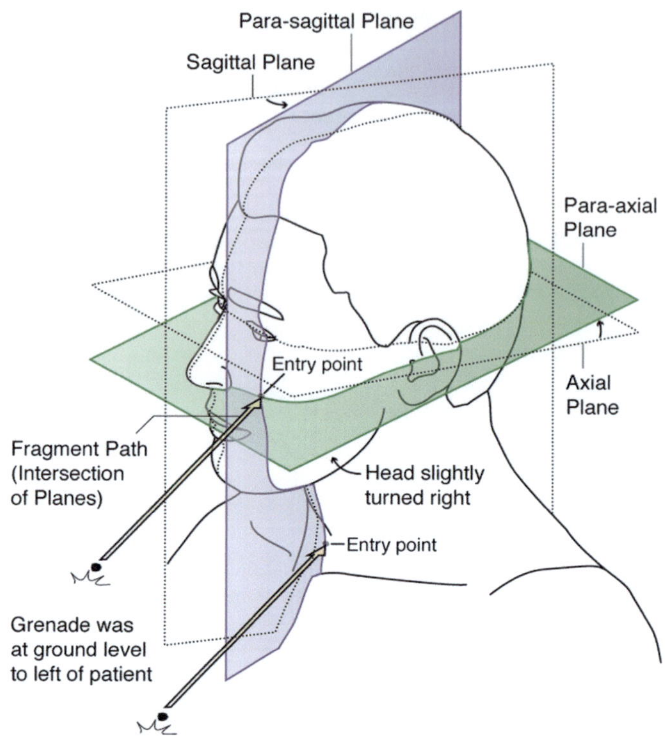

Fig. 5.31 This similar drawing now includes the second fragment, best explained and identified by finding the first fragment and trajectory. Reprinted with permission from Military Medicine: International Journal of AMSUS

Fig. 5.66 for sniper/range, and Fig. 5.67 for target in controlled environment using laser range finders and clinometers for accurate angles. Figure 5.68 shows how realistic the synthetic anatomic models respond to gunshot wounds. The appearance is similar to what I have experienced in Iraq. Figure 5.69 shows measuring the angle with the PACS angle tool on a para-coronal image aligned along the wound path. Initial data show that the angles measured by radiologists are within 5° of actual angles shot.

5.10 Description of Mapped Planes

After completion of construction of the planes, finding the trajectory of the missile path, the radiologist can better explain the involvement of surrounding anatomic structures such as vessels, nerves, etc. This is paramount to immediate damage control trauma surgery. Existing planar orientation boxes on some PACS systems

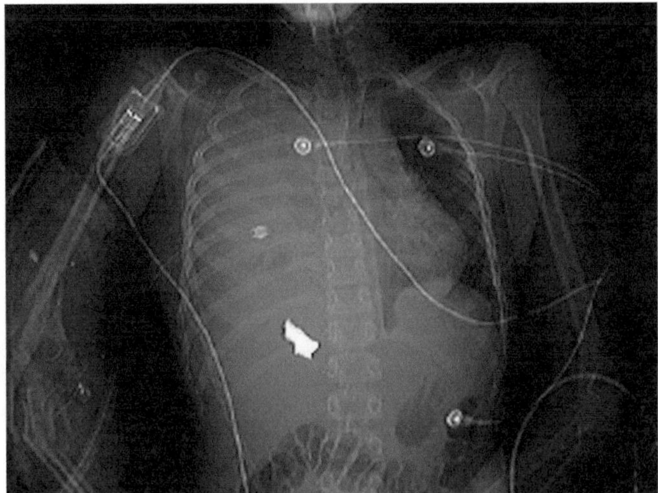

Fig. 5.32 Frontal chest CT scout shows a large metallic fragment in the RUQ. In addition to the large hemothorax on the right, there is tracheal deviation from increasing pressure in the left hemithorax from bleeding on the right. Diaphragm disruption is suspected based on fragment location and entry clinically. Note fracture of right humerus with associated fragments near elbow from fragment entry angle on an axial plane. Reprinted with permission from Military Medicine: International Journal of AMSUS

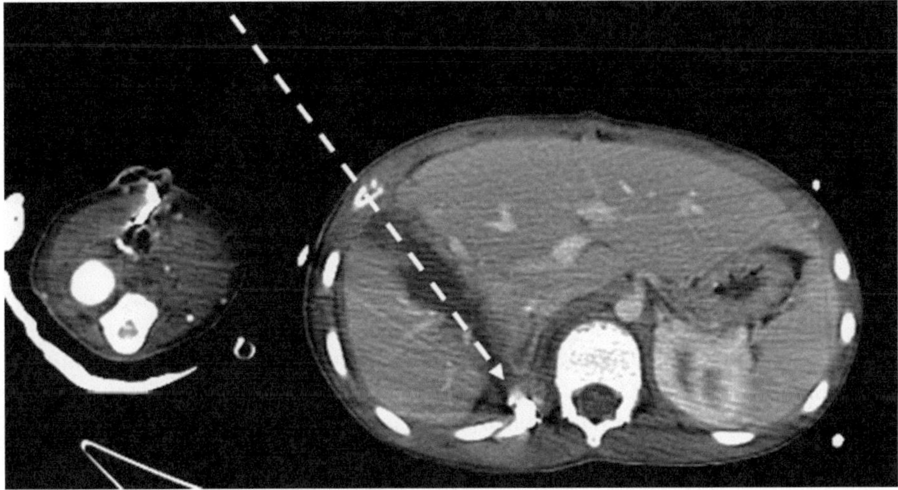

Fig. 5.33 Para-axial slice showing path of projectile (*dotted arrow*) from a blast fragment going through the liver from anterior right toward midline posterior. Additional metallic remnants in the right arm anteriorly support the entry direction and planar trajectory. Reprinted with permission from Military Medicine: International Journal of AMSUS

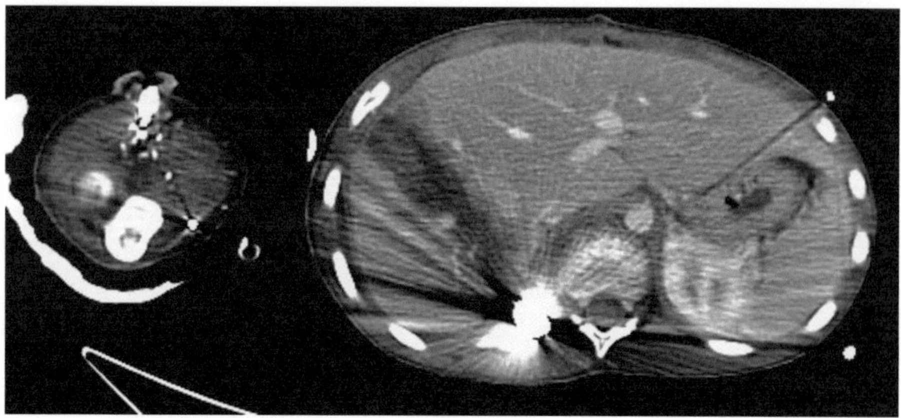

Fig. 5.34 A lower Para-axial MPR showing the large fragments and destruction possible with these traveling at high speed

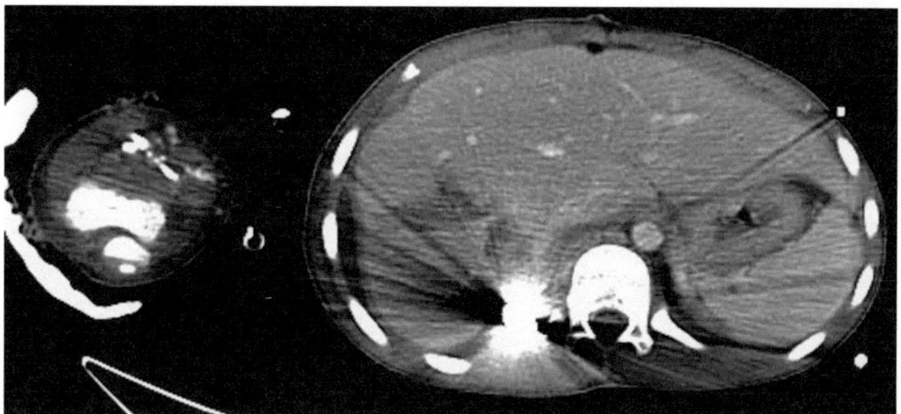

Fig. 5.35 A lower Para-axial MPR showing the large fragments and destruction possible with these traveling at high speed

attempt to show the plane of reformation, however, the authors believe that real-time animation models would be more effective in helping radiologists orient surgeons and other providers. This system, once integrated into reading workstations should immediately paint the picture in the users mind as to the exact orientation of the plane displayed. The grenade injury described above should highlight this application well. Such system allows for the description of any complex plane, intersecting line, or even point. This has application beyond military and penetrating trauma in that many other specialties, modalities, and medical sciences deal with descriptive planes, lines, or point locations.

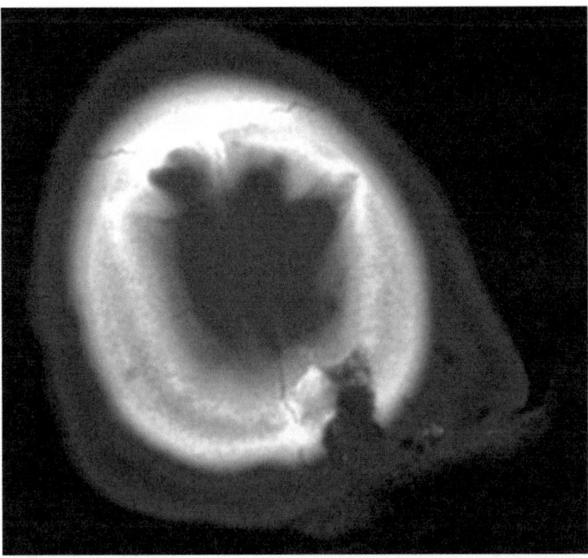

Fig. 5.36 Axial CT of high convexity of patient with GSW grazing top of skull. Note the keyhole shape (note that keyhole upside down) to the defect indicated shot came from behind and slightly above patient

Fig. 5.37 Axial CT of brain showing acute bleed from indriven bone fragments from same patient, indicating severity of injury. The wound can appear trivial clinically, however, the keyhole shape should alert radiologists to alert ED physicians of urgent need for immediate neurosurgical involvement. Reprinted with permission from Military Medicine: International Journal of AMSUS

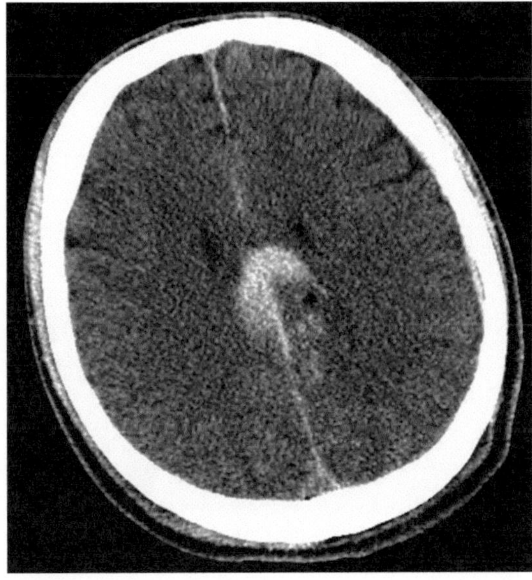

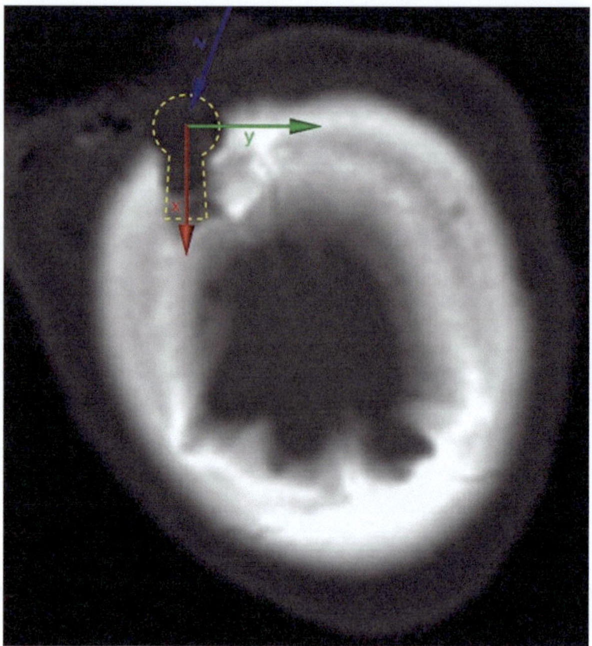

Fig. 5.38 The same high convexity axial CT, now turned upside down to show upright orientation of keyhole for instructional purposes. Reprinted with permission from Military Medicine: International Journal of AMSUS

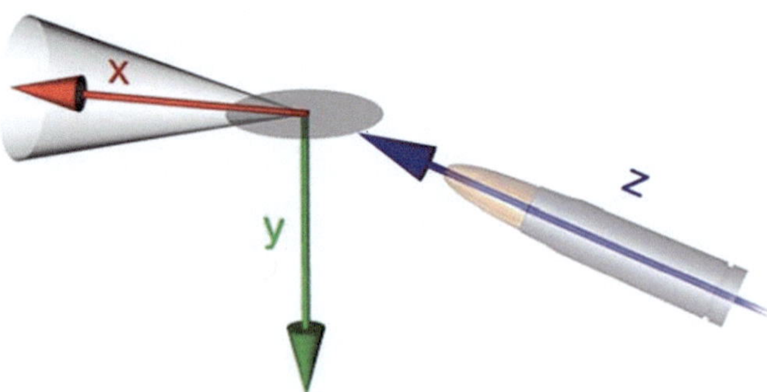

Fig. 5.39 Artist drawing of resultant force vectors of bullet striking (disregard shell of bullet) curved bone (these can also occur to curved hollow long bones such as femur). Reprinted with permission from Military Medicine: International Journal of AMSUS

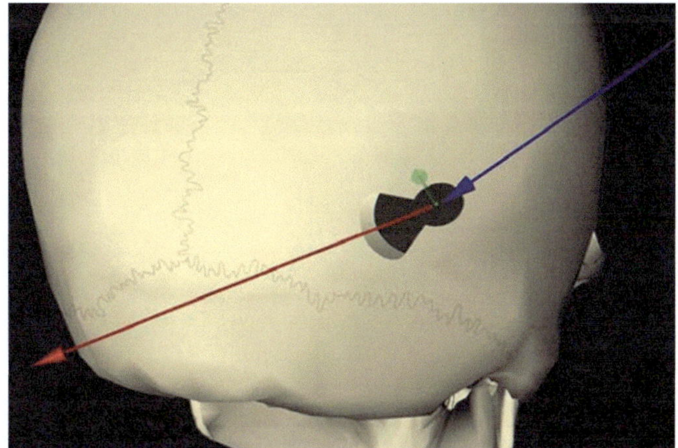

Fig. 5.40 Drawing of skull with different (from the patient highlighted here)) angle of bullet trajectory. This bullet traveled from anterior-superior toward posterior-inferior. Blue arrow shows trajectory before impact ("entrance"), and green arrow shows direction of indriven bone fragments (the "projectile"). Note beveling of "exit" wound (*red arrow*). Reprinted with permission from Military Medicine: International Journal of AMSUS

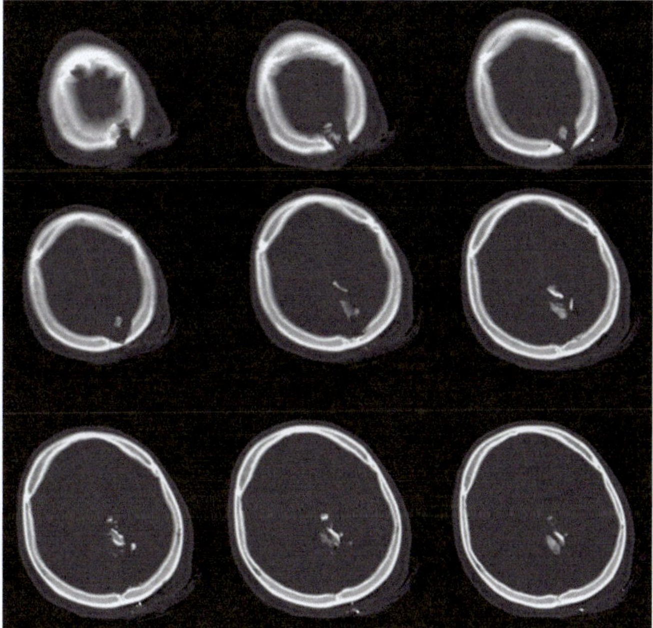

Fig. 5.41 Series of axial CT in bone windows highlighting the indriven bone fragments that cause the brain damage. Reprinted with permission from Military Medicine: International Journal of AMSUS

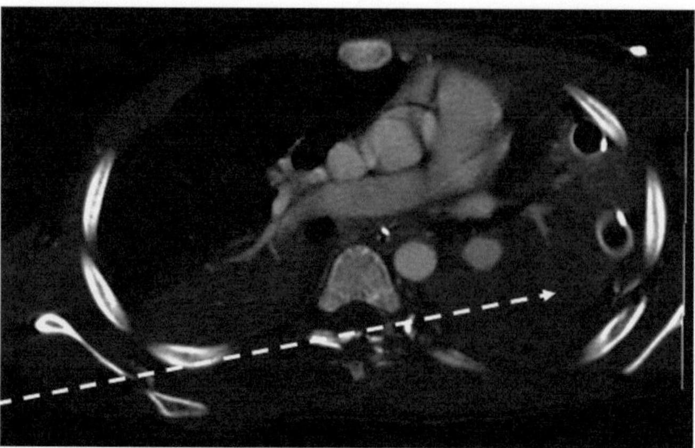

Fig. 5.42 CT axial bone windows show the wound path of this GSW victim across his right scapula, through his thoracic spinal elements traversing the left lung and out through his left ribs evidenced by fractures. Fractures and damage along the path help determine the wound path and resultant trajectory

5.11 Further Quantification and Application of Coordinate System Relative, to a Standard Reference

The following takes the complex planes one step further in quantifying fragment orientations and specific locations. A reference point was chosen with the following background to support this decision. Spinal curvatures and structure–function relationships utilize planes and plumb lines to describe and quantify stability [26]. The sagittal vertical axis (SVA), for example, is defined by the C7 plumb line on a lateral radiograph and is used to evaluate the sagittal profile of patients with scoliosis. The C7 plumb line should ideally intersect the posterior superior corner of the sacrum (PSCS), and is termed neutral. Anterior/posterior (horizontal) displacement of the C7 plumb line from the PSCS is termed positive if anterior, and negative if posterior.

I chose the PSCS as the center point for a few reasons: it is a consistent region near the skin surface posterioly and previously described as an anatomic/physiologic landmark. Also, in severe combat casualty care, it is my experience that this region is maintained and consistent in surviving combat casualties. See Fig. 5.70 for a drawing of the C7 plumb line to include the PSCS. It is the intersection of the SVA and the mid sagittal planes that define the proposed reference point. Figure 5.71 shows example application of specification of fragment locations from angle and magnitude from the reference point. Figure 5.72 shows how 3D localization can be represented by a vector ray (in degrees) with magnitude (cm) on the x-, y-, and z-axis. Once the process is automated to identify, quantify, and localize spatial coordinates accurately, prior datasets already dictated can be analyzed for fragment specific patterns from an epidemiological perspective. In addition, automated detection and

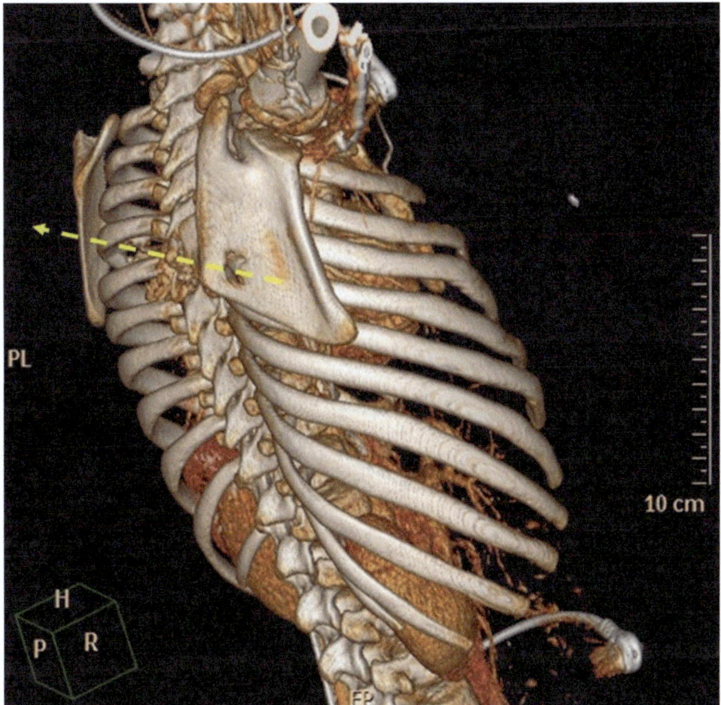

Fig. 5.43 Volume rendered 3D image showing pathway through scapula and ribs. In a similar, however, much less severe case, a bullet entered the left back of another patient, perforated the left scapula, tangentially skimmed a rib resulting in a focal contusion of the left lung, just missing spine, before finally lodging between the right scapula and the ribs (see Figs. 5.44 and 5.45). The bullet skimming the left ribs also caused a localized hematoma to the left upper lobe lung

localization reporting can supplement the radiologist report, saving radiologists time, while providing more objective data.

To validate consistent localization of points in three dimensions, I put together a CT phantom using a plastic tub, wooden dowels with nail heads (stem trimmed) at the tips at random locations in x, y, and z planes (see Fig. 5.73). These points were measured by three independent observers on the phantom itself, then by radiologists on CT. Preliminary work is showing consistent measurements to within millimeters. This will be compared to patient data and movement of fragments over time. Missile embolus and migration was already described earlier in this chapter.

Determining and describing trajectory angles with standardized terminology and retained fragments using standard polar coordinates may help the study of individual incidents as well as for an epidemiologic baseline in recording and comparing gunshot and blast trajectories for years to come. The proposed systems have some limitations in that the plane description is new, our terminology based on available literature and not validated beyond experience in a combat hospital. In addition, some patients suffering GSW or blast injury have complex paths that

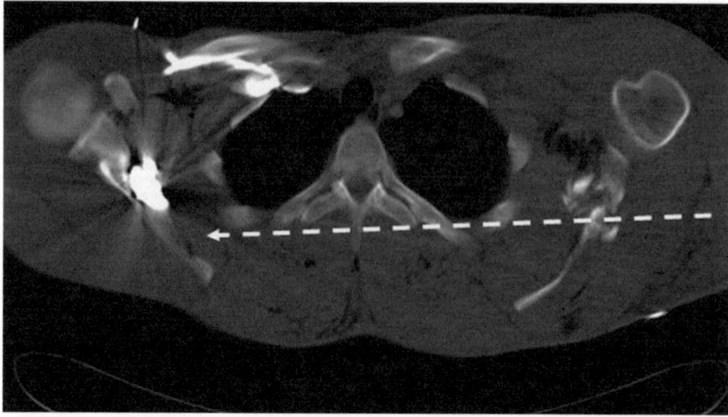

Fig. 5.44 Another patient with a GSW across the back, this time through the left scapula, skimming the left ribs and resting just anterior and medial to the right scapula

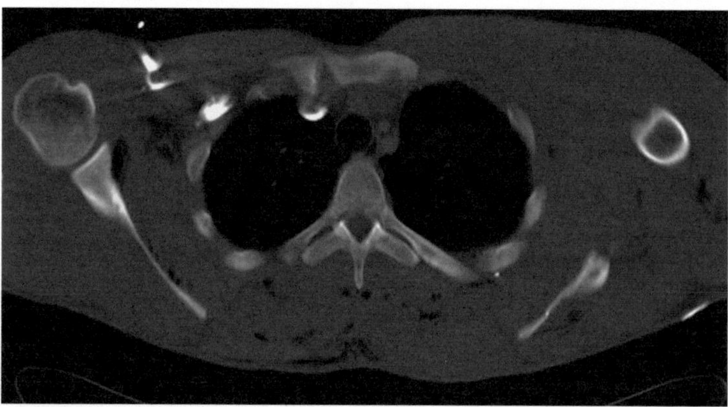

Fig. 5.45 Axial CT bone windows slightly lower than Fig. 5.44 demonstrating a tiny metallic fragment just posterior to the left posterior ribs. This highlights how using all clues can help determine wound path. Not the extensive subcutaneous emphysema highlighting the wound path as well

may have chaotic pathways or ricochets that do not lend themselves to analysis described here. Complex ricochets were much less common in our population, however. In addition, there seems to be a superior to inferior analytical probability relationship in that the more superior a pathway, the more probably a trajectory can be determined. Further research is needed to test quantification and reproducibility.

Not all ballistic missiles travel through tissues in a predictable manner. For example, some explosions result in fragments that are too numerous to count or

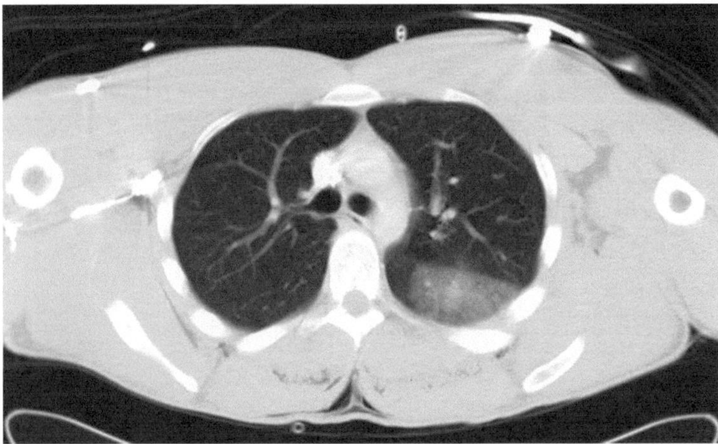

Fig. 5.46 Axial CT lung windows showing a wedge-shaped consolidation of the LUL posteriorly representing a lung contusion from the impact of the bullet

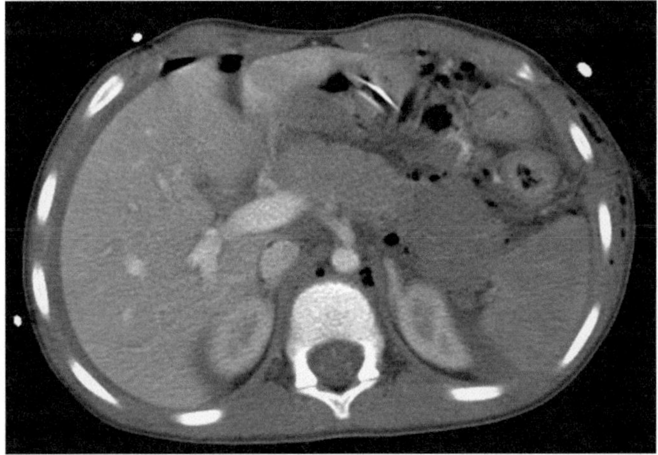

Fig. 5.47 Axial post IV contrast CT of a child that suffered extensive organ damage from a blast fragment. Note the peritoneal fluid representing blood, intra peritoneal air and retrocrural air, devascularized spleen, and pancreatic hematoma. Reprinted with permission from Military Medicine: International Journal of AMSUS

evaluate effectively. By determining reporting size thresholds used in virtual autopsy, protocols on reporting can allow simplification of otherwise complex situations as to not get bogged down trying to report on hundreds of fragments.

These situations could result in increased time to analyze and post-process images, possibly negatively impacting efficiency. Established realistic protocols

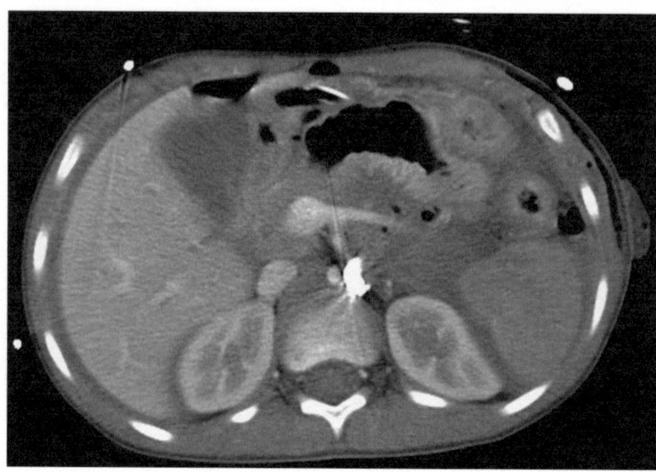

Fig. 5.48 Axial CT through the level of the retained blast fragment showing close proximity to the aorta, just above the renal arteries. Note again extensive peritoneal fluid with sparing of major vasculature. Reprinted with permission from Military Medicine: International Journal of AMSUS

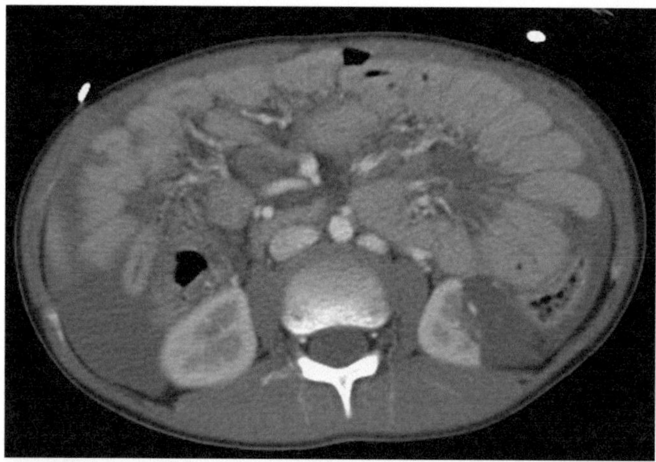

Fig. 5.49 CT more inferior showing damage to left kidney, some subcutaneous air in left soft tissues, and extensive peritoneal fluid. Generalized shock bowel is present, however, the IVC is maintained due to aggressive hydration since just after the injury. Reprinted with permission from Military Medicine: International Journal of AMSUS

will guide radiologists to most effectively analyze the majority of cases and know when exact determination of peppered fragments (for example) are just not possible to effectively record.

The authors are currently working on development of systems to help delineate trajectories of penetrating wounds from blast injuries using an automated computer

Fig. 5.50 Coronal MIP showing the fragment orientation to the aorta. MIPS can be helpful in showing orientation, however, should not be relied upon for determining active bleeding or other precise localization. Reprinted with permission from Military Medicine: International Journal of AMSUS

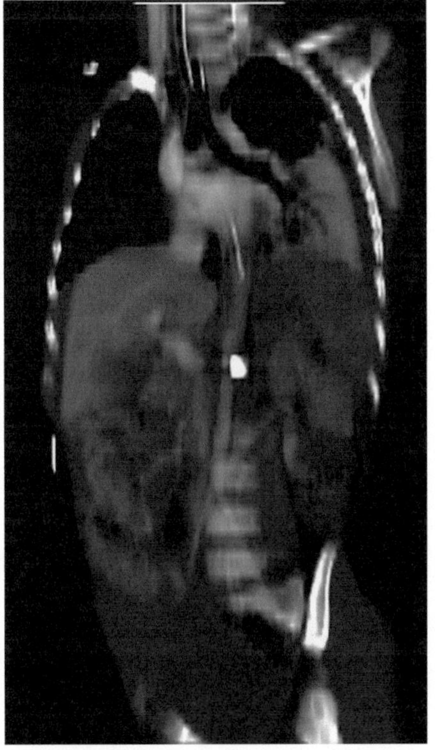

Fig. 5.51 Para-coronal MIP showing the blast fragment pathway from left flank through kidney, tail of pancreas, and final resting spot near aorta. These help trauma surgeons find the fragment with least amount of exploration and least surprise. Reprinted with permission from Military Medicine: International Journal of AMSUS

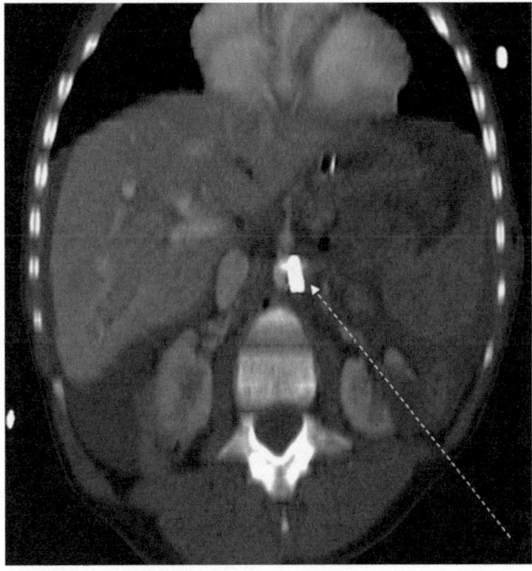

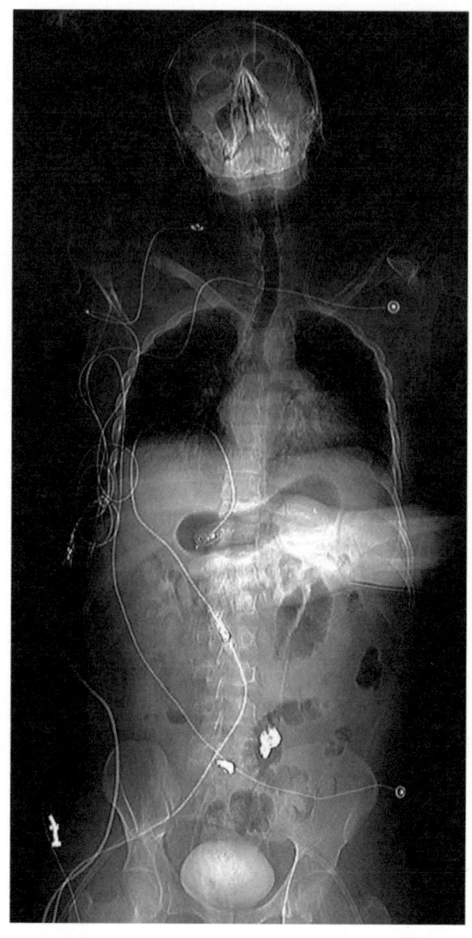

Fig. 5.52 CT delayed scout of two large metal fragments in mid-lower abdomen. There was no evidence of ureter involvement on delayed imaging. Reprinted with permission from Military Medicine: International Journal of AMSUS

assisted plane derived from pattern recognition. Recent advancements will allow precise automated recording of trajectories to help individual patients by a standard reporting system that can follow war casualties through the echelons of care. Automated analysis of remaining fragments of wounded soldiers for example, will streamline the otherwise tedious job describing these subjectively, with consistent accepted coordinates. It is hoped in our current projects to validate 1 cm location accuracy in x, y, z planes (ray and magnitude) and 5° angular resolution on trajectory angles.

Once a ballistic localization and planar lexicon is agreed upon and algorithms are developed, automated quantification systems will allow expeditious accountability of all fragments and recorded trajectories of all wounded warriors in a

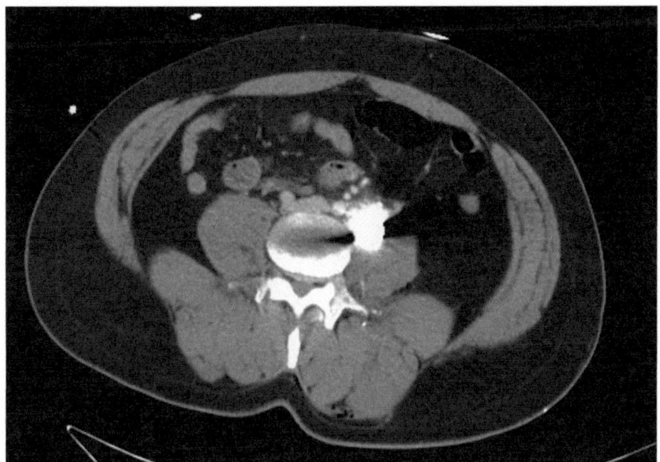

Fig. 5.53 This large fragment lies within the left psoas. The reformatted images helped demonstrate the lack of intraperitoneal component, i.e., this fragment path was shown to be mostly muscular. The fractured transverse process, subcutaneous air and soft tissue aberration were all supporting evidence of the missile path. Reprinted with permission from Military Medicine: International Journal of AMSUS

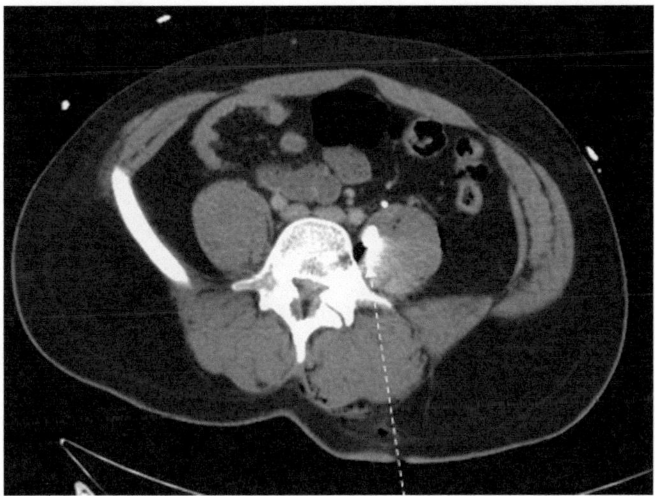

Fig. 5.54 Although the fragment size, irregularity and location appears concerning when not considering trajectory as it lies near major vessels, when surgeons were convinced it came through the back and not traversing cord or vessels, this patient was re-triaged at a lower priority since other casualties were in need of immediate surgery at the same time

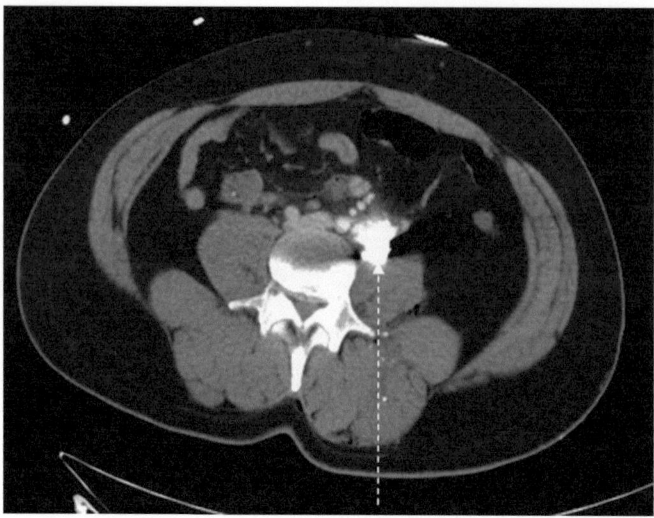

Fig. 5.55 Note metallic peppered fragments in left paravertebral musculature (along the arrow) supporting the trajectory path

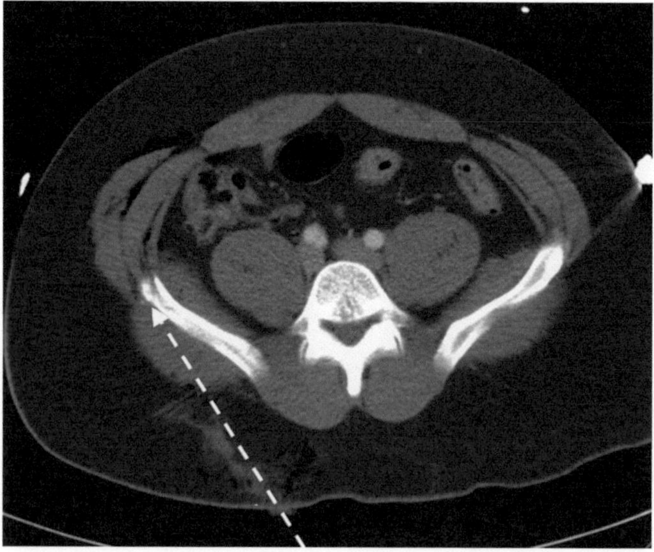

Fig. 5.56 This superior para-axial CT reformat illustrates a perforating fragment that entered to the back, traveled through the right posterior flank avoiding the peritoneum and ricocheted off the right iliac wing. Note small nondisplaced fracture of anterior iliac wing. Reprinted with permission from Military Medicine: International Journal of AMSUS

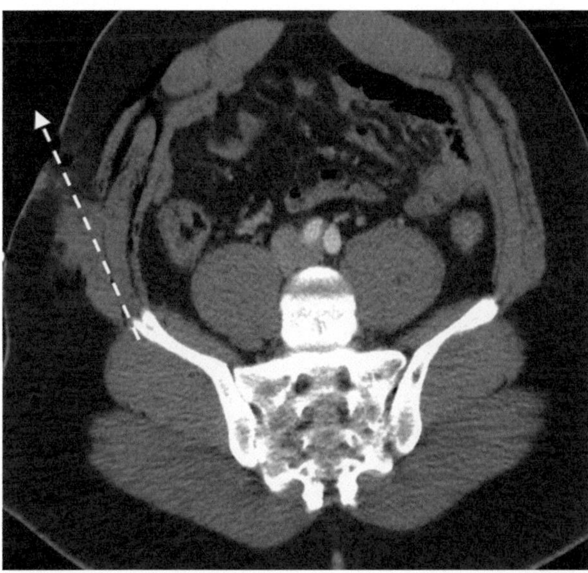

Fig. 5.57 Upward angled para-axial CT reformat showing the exit path verified by exit wound (skin near arrow). Multi-planar reformation showed that the path was deflected superiorly (dotted arrow) after striking the right iliac wing. This required two reformats, both in para-axial orientations. Reprinted with permission from Military Medicine: International Journal of AMSUS

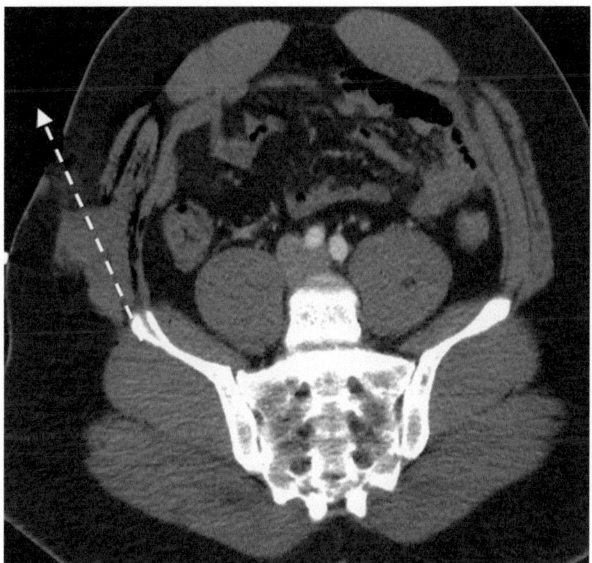

Fig. 5.58 Another upward angled para-axial CT reformat further supporting exit path. Reprinted with permission from Military Medicine: International Journal of AMSUS

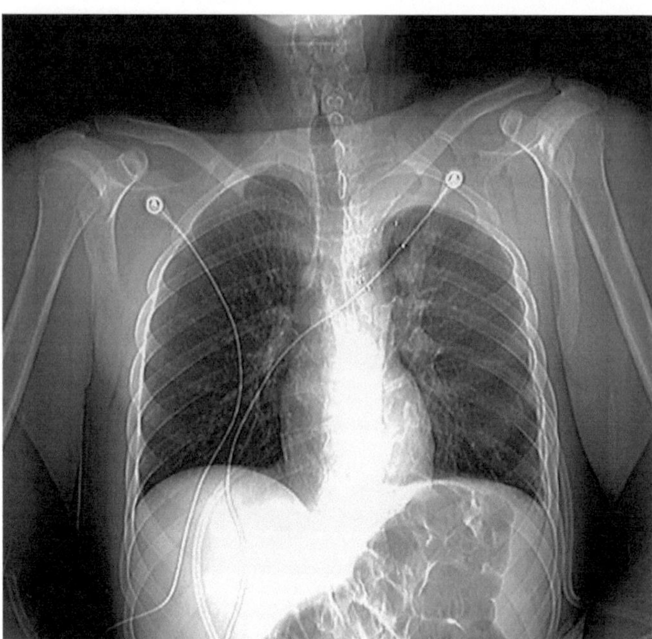

Fig. 5.59 Scout CT substitute for chest radiograph demonstrates obliteration of normal left subclavian stripe and thickening of the left apical region consistent with localized hemothorax from GSW to the left chest. Some overall haziness to the left thorax is from superimposing hemothorax and decreased overall volume of left lung. There are some retained fragments, localized consolidation from the wound path in the perforating injury (entrance anterior, exit posterior)

consistent recording fashion. In addition to helping each soldier, sailor, airman, and marine exposed to blast or gunshot, a standard and accurate database will establish epidemiological patterns forming a research baseline for years to come.

Included here several cases of penetrating injuries from combat hospitals highlighting wound ballistics and trajectory analysis, while introducing descriptions of complex anatomic planes now possible with advanced imaging in combat. We have shown how application of complex planes can accurately describe wound trajectories in a more quantitative and repeatable fashion. This descriptive system should enhance communication between radiologists and other physicians. Furthermore, standardized and quantitative descriptions of trajectories based on use of complex planes and coordinates now possible with MDCT introduced here may help in long-term study of gunshot and blast injuries.

Using a standardized plane-based data acquisition and analysis approach, we will be able to precisely locate a fragment, estimate its size, and delineate its three-dimensional shape, which provides guidance for triage nurses, trauma

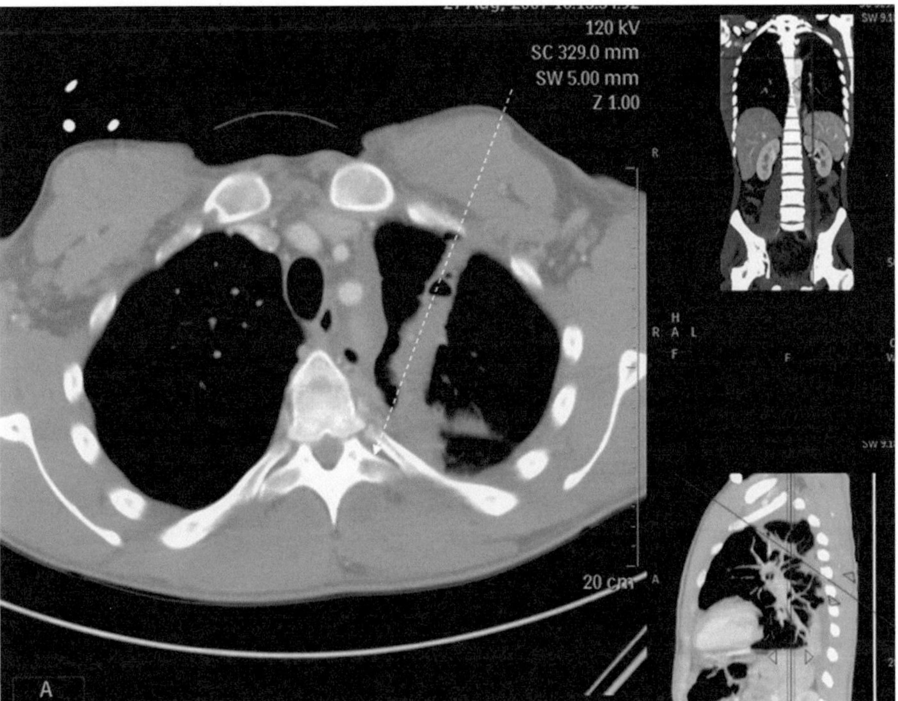

Fig. 5.60 Para-axial reformation of ballistic trajectory showing small air-fluid level in resultant cavity, contusion, and associated hemothorax. The coronal and para-sagittal scout reference images help orient providers to the extent of the missile pathway. Also note the superior to inferior trajectory (*red line* on para-axial image *lower right*), and the posterior (dependent) localized hemothorax

surgeons, and follow-up evaluations through the echelons of care. This will have obvious implications for the long-term prognosis and follow-up of such injuries. Precise planar description of missile paths will help standardize communication between radiologists, trauma surgeons, and ED physicians. Our complex-plane-base approach will also enhance incident analysis in forensic medicine including sniper attacks, military combat firefights, and random gunshot injuries.

Knowing the para-axial or otherwise complex planes of known fragments may help solve for unknown fragments by keeping the same para-axial orientation during interpretation. In addition, consistent reporting, standard nomenclature, and possibly quantification should allow for more descriptive recording of GSW and blast fragments, especially since many of the original image datasets are often lost during transition of wounded warriors through the echelons of care. More research is needed in this specific area.

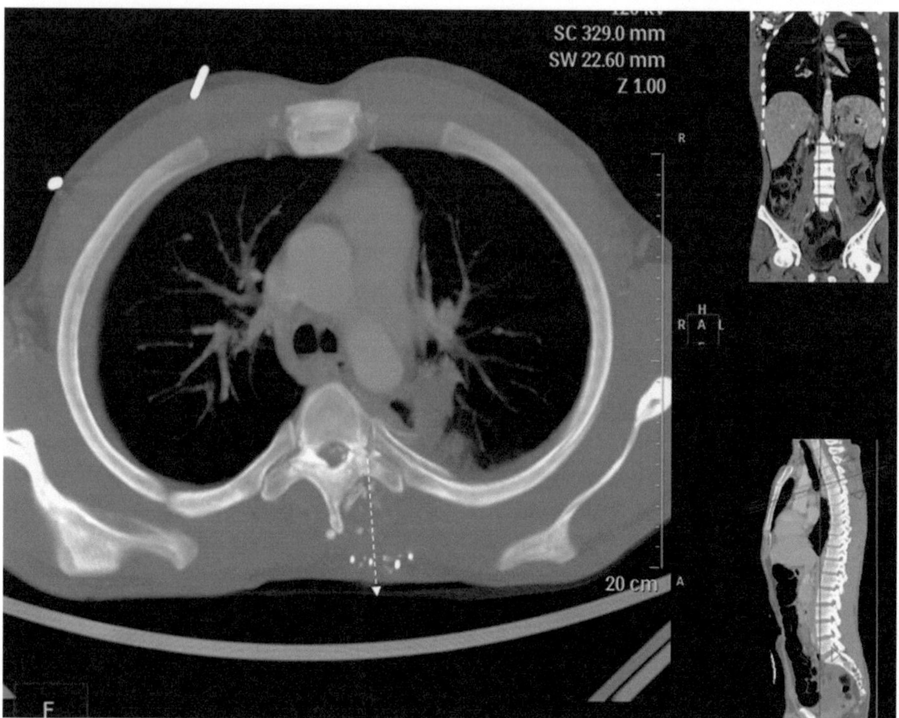

Fig. 5.61 This para-axial MIP shows the bone fragments dispersed after the bullet hitting lateral aspect of the bony spinal elements. Note rib alignment indicating downsloping para-axial orientation, hence upward deflection of bullet after impact with spine. The arrow shows the ricocheted trajectory

5.12   Decision Support Tools, Expert Systems

Online decision support tools seem to be on the rise. When I was at the Uniform Services University, I developed a teaching tool called RoboChest (from Adobe® RoboHelp®) built with directory structures to allow students and residents to dig as deep as they like on an area of interest in the chest X-ray. It attempts to impart to the students a systematic methodology of evaluating abnormalities shown on chest X-rays, the most common type of medical imaging performed, and interpreting those findings in light of the clinical setting.

The chunked information in a structured lexicon is designed to link from a larger project called "ChestWeb," an expert system to help guide image interpretation. This content follows the organization of how material is presented to medical students at the USU's F. Edward Hebert School of Medicine.

I believe this type of approach is effective and efficient in teaching principles of radiographic image interpretation.

Fig. 5.62 Para-sagittal reformat along the angled thoracic wound path showing initial downward trajectory (from a sniper, since anterior to posterior, and superior to inferior), until impacting vertebral elements, then ricocheting superiorly (*shorter dotted arrow*) for a more superior exit than expected. Note the moderate amount of hemothorax dependently

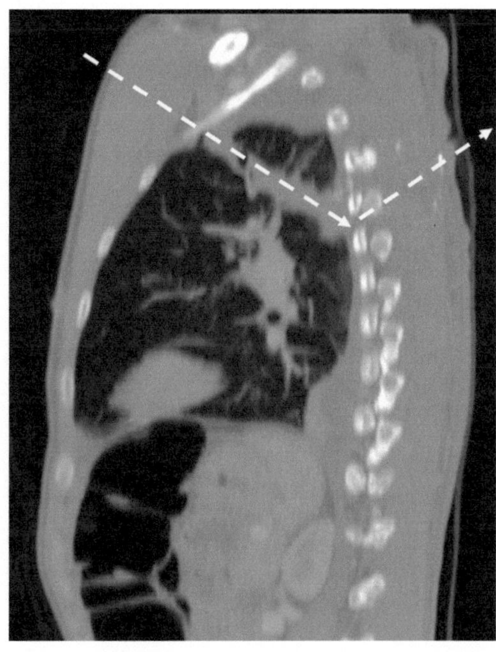

Fig. 5.63 Para-axial CT bone windows showing the sniper bullet's trajectory though the spinal canal at C4. Note retained bullet near the skin surface on the patients right

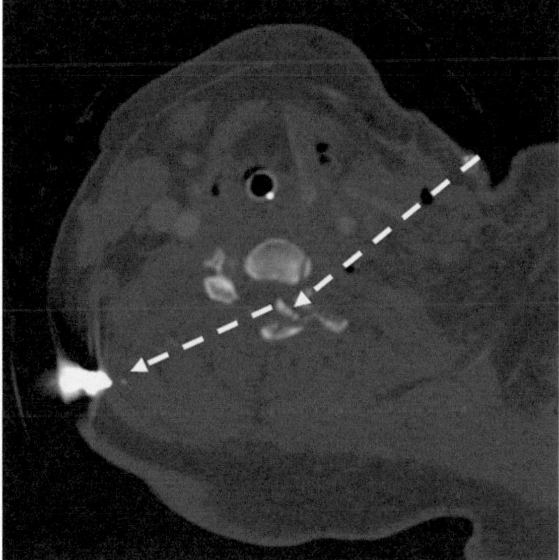

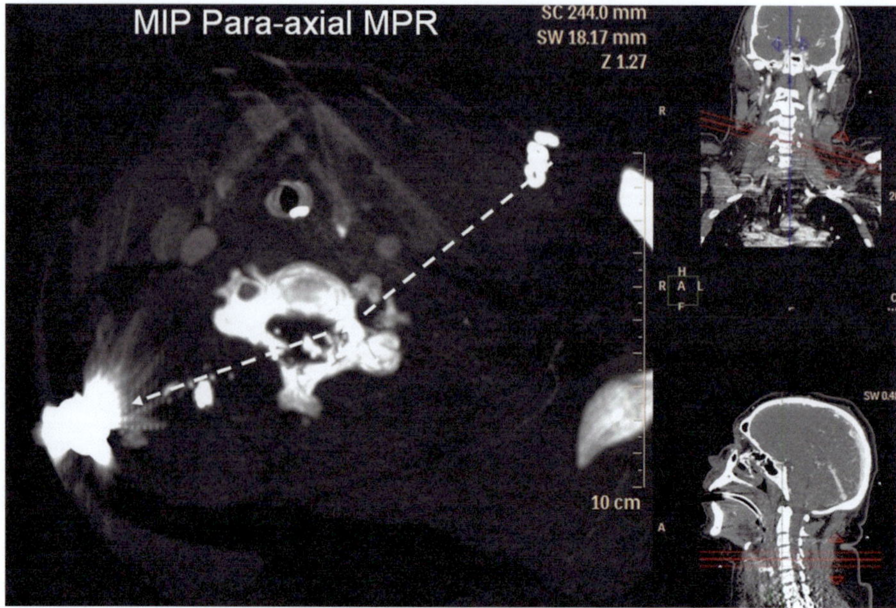

Fig. 5.64 Para-axial MIP reformat verifying the sniper bullet's trajectory though the spinal canal at C4. The fractured vertebra and remaining bullet indicate the slight deflection of the pathway after impacting the bone

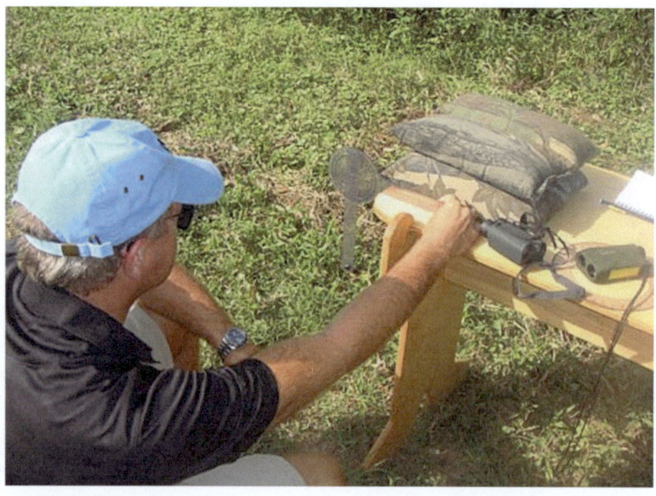

Fig. 5.65 In this figure, I am determining the angle of the sniper bench with a clinometer. We also measured the zeroed-out barrel of the weapon just prior to shooting downrange at the target (Photo by Dr. Mike Frew)

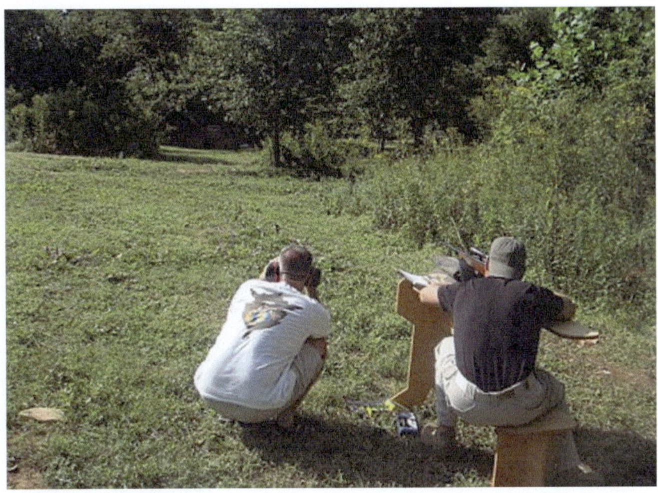

Fig. 5.66 This photo shows the sniper aiming at the synthetic targets downrange. The spotter is using binoculars to evaluate accuracy of the shot, and a camera is mounted on a tripod near the target for slow motion analysis (Photo by Dr. Les Folio)

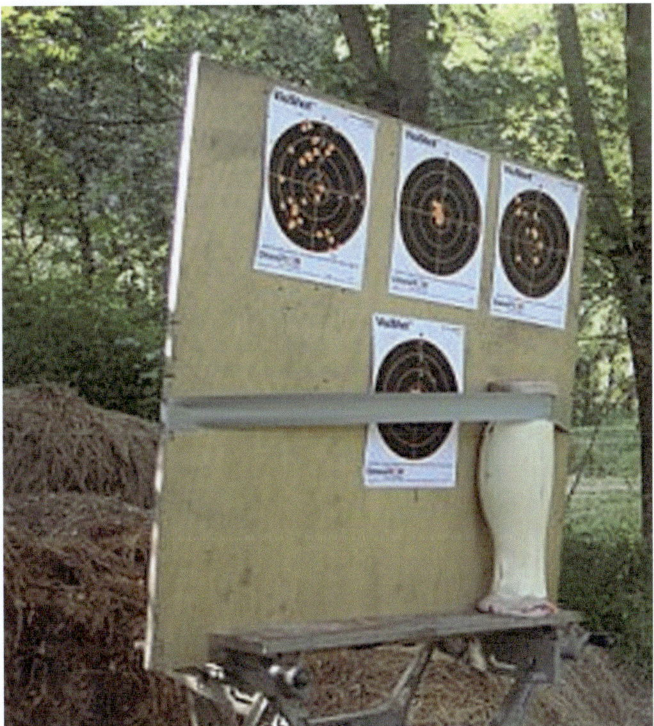

Fig. 5.67 The anatomic ballistic model was fastened to a stable bench as the target. Various known sniping angles were accomplished (Photo by Dr. Les Folio)

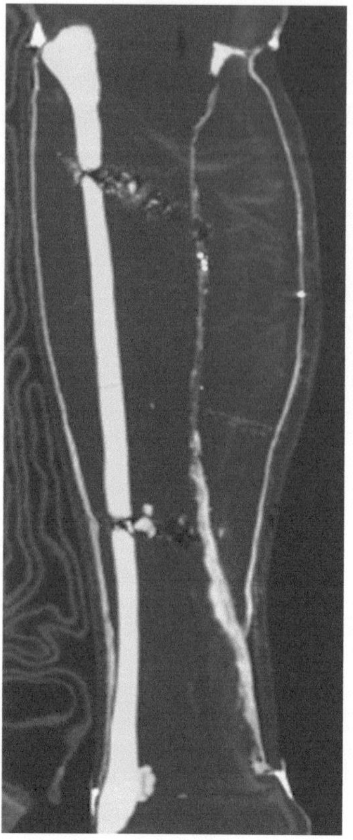

Fig. 5.68 MD CT para-coronal reformation along the path of a 40° trajectory. The facial planes are as dense as the synthetic bone because this particular model was used for training emergent faciitomies for deploying military surgeons

The goal of these systems is for medical students to reproducibly describe radiographic abnormalities detected on plain film CXRs. The lexicon is designed to provide the students with clinically significant differentiation of abnormalities detected. The content is chunked in a directory structure that relates specific combinations of distinct radiographic findings to classes/groupings based on findings.

5.13   Telehealth on the Battlefield

Teleradiology is an important part of casualty management up the echelons of care. It is imperative that image data movement, archiving, and matching textual data is moved along with the patients that are transported to follow-on medical centers. An overview of the status of teleradiology was presented at a conference in 2007.

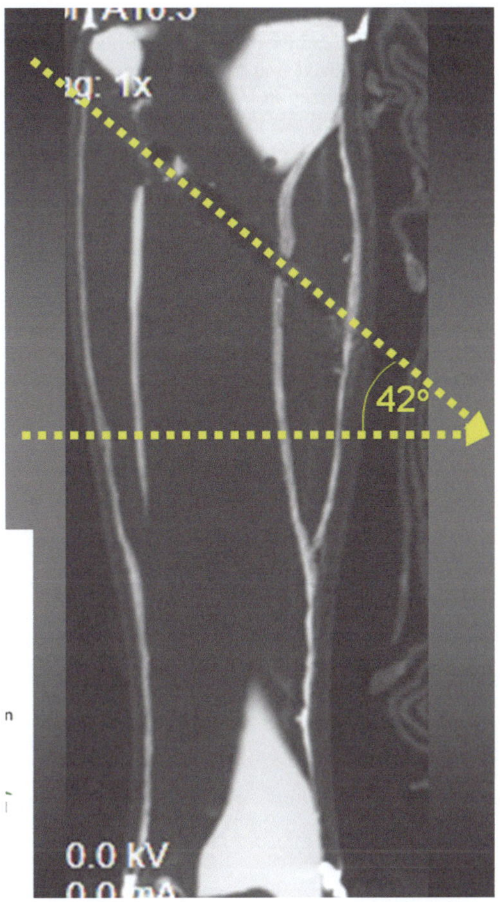

Fig. 5.69 Another MD CT para-coronal reformation reconstructed along a wound path showing how the PACS angle tool can easily determine the angle of the sniping

Additionally, more information on the triservice status on telehealth can be found in Military Medical Technology [27]. I also have led teams into Iraq and other countries to help develop teleradiology issues [28].

As is often the case in combat medicine, interim solutions proliferate as providers do whatever they can to best treat their patients. This includes assembling montages of CT images to send via e-mail using mp4 [29]. Another technology that helps display more efficiently and quickly is Universal Trauma Window [30]. This is a technological solution to the Damage Control Radiology mentioned previously in this book.

Some practitioners take digital photos of dermatology lesions for consults on perplexing cases when no dermatologist is available. These solutions are novel, secure, and compliant, but they demonstrate the need for a more uniform solution that can be replicated.

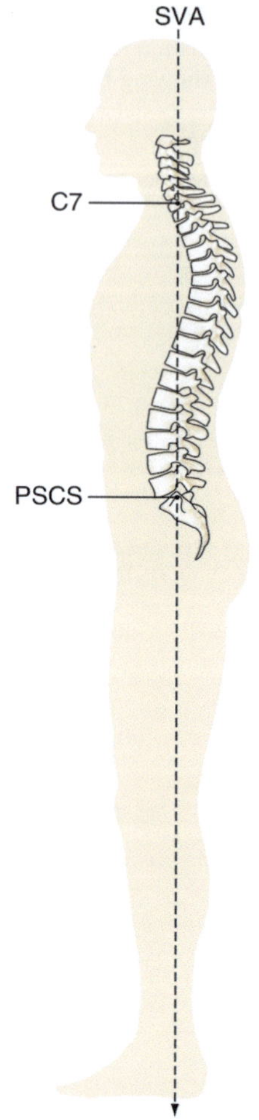

Fig. 5.70 Drawing of the spine from the side showing how the PSCS is used for postural exams and research. Prior reference to this consistently localized area led to selection for a standard reference point for fragment localization

Some evolving solutions include online health vaults that are being studied with the US Army [31]. These could answer the RIS-HIS interoperability issues using the compression and window technologies described above.

Finally, one technology that may have application in blast and ballistic imaging is total body scanning. The StatScan by Lodox [32] can obtain AP and lateral plain radiography of the entire body in seconds. Experience at UMM Baltimore Shock Trauma is promising [33].

In summary, recent advances on the battlefield have contributed significantly to record survival rates. While difficult to attribute each advance with actual percentage of increased lives saved, it is obvious that all of these advances have contributed their part to the heroic results combat medics and those supporting them have achieved.

Fig. 5.71 Artist drawing demonstrating how fragments can be consistently localized in 3D using the reference point for epidemiologic tracking over time. A fragment score can be assigned as well for the individual

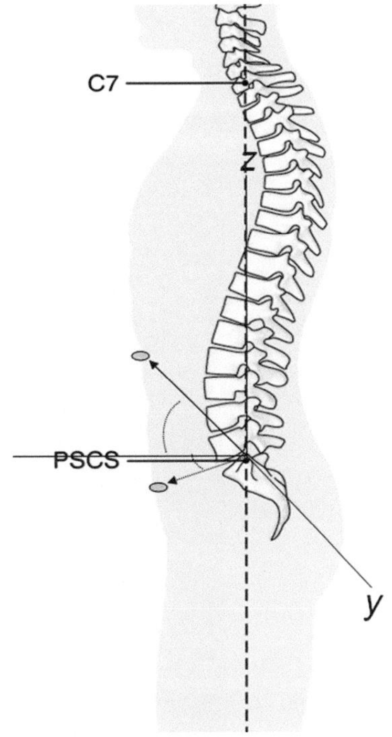

Fig. 5.72 A basic vector magnitude using x, y, z coordinates can be assigned to each fragment for precise localization that can be added to patient's records and for future consistent data mining

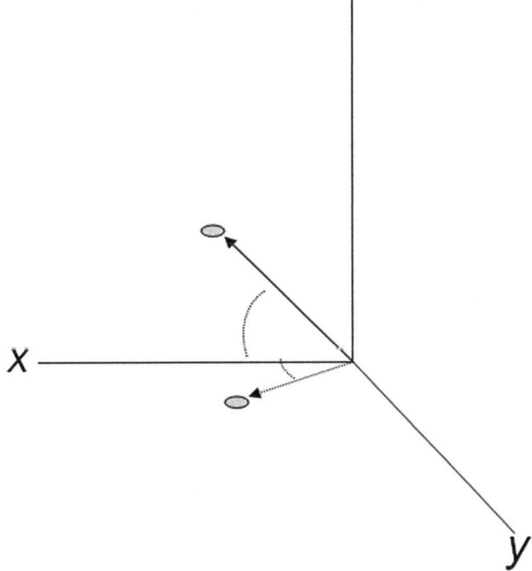

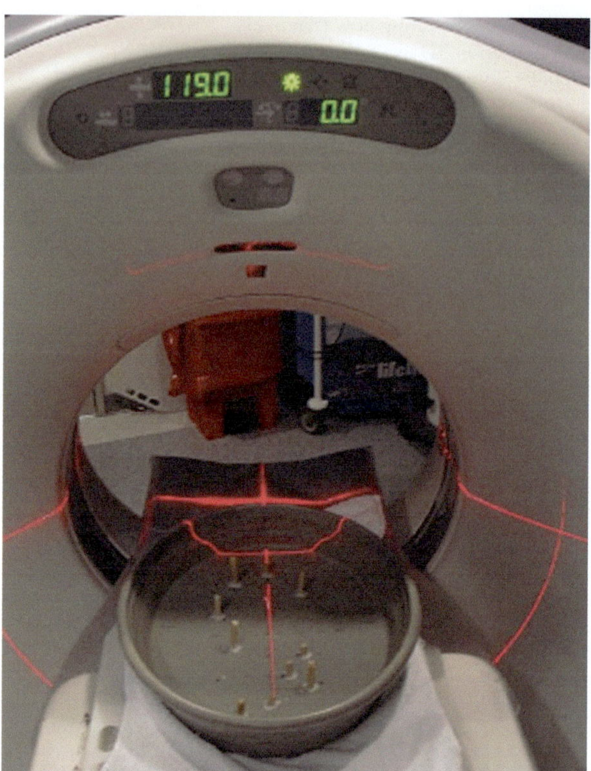

Fig. 5.73 The blast belly phantom I created for one study to allow measurements of 3D localization of simulated blast fragments. This was filled with water for attenuation fidelity and will be measured by radiologists for accuracy

Acknowledgments I would like to thank the following individuals for making this chapter possible. Dr. Rolf Bunger, for mentoring me on the trajectory analysis and APS concept. He encouraged me to further develop this work as he saw the potential clinical and public health impact. It was his idea to establish a reference point, whether it be the one that prevails over time or not, get that point and show that we can localize consistently. I would also like to thank Tatjana Fischer from the Technical University of Munich, Germany for choosing me as her mentor for her Ph.D. in APS and ballistic trajectory analysis. We succeeded in validating APS and that trajectories can be determined and calculated in actual combat casualties. To Lt Chris Backus USU class of 2010 for his piloting background and stimulating completion of the complex plane descriptions when he was a second year medical student. Also thanks to Sofia Echelmeyer for her excellent illustrations. To Gerd Frankfurter for brainstorming with me on the field ballistic study design. To Bill Knepshield, CEO of Operative Experiences, Inc. for donating the anatomic leg simulators. To Michael Frew, MD, and David Cruea for the sniping expertise and range. I would also like to thank Israel Felix, RT, and David Stancil; RT for working with us on getting high quality CTs of the legs and blast belly phantom. Thanks also to Dr. Andy Dwyer for helping with the Cartesian and trajectory calculator. Anna Grefe for her consultation in right triangles and 3D coordinates. Photos by Dominik Usling.

References

1. Abrames EL, Chen SR, Jones W, Folio L. Traumatic carotid pseudoaneurysm post gun shot wound to the head/neck. Mil Med. 2008 May; 173(5):xv-xvi.
2. Backus C, Folio L. Lung laceration with active bleeding, contusion and hemothorax. Mil Med. 2008 Aug; 173(8):xv-xvi.
3. Albery WB. Acceleration in other axes affects _Gz tolerance: dynamic centrifuge simulation of agile flight. Aviat Space Environ Med. 2004; 75(1):1–6.
4. Gao X, Xue Z, Xing J, Lee DY, Gottschalk SM, Heslop HE, Bollard CM, Wong ST. Computer-assisted quantitative evaluation of therapeutic responses for lymphoma using serial PET/CT imaging. Acad Radiol. 2010 Apr; 17(4):479–488.
5. Gel'fand IM, Glagoleva EG, Kirllov AA. The method of coordinates. p.52. Available at: http://books.google.com/books?id=InstSVAf5wC&pg=PA56&lpg=PA56&dq=three-dimensional+plane+x+y+z&source=web&ots=625PBbcCGw&sig=pzyf1SxTKb4m4CbXqZkMPtcot-k&hl=en&sa=X&oi=book_result&resnum=10&ct=result#PPA52,M1 (Accessed on Jan 2009).
6. Bruckner BA, Norman M, Scott BG. CT tractogram: technique for demonstrating tangential bullet trajectories. J Trauma. 2006; 60(6):1362–1363.
7. Shogan P, Fischer T, Bunger R, Frew M, Provenzale J, Folio L. Anatomic positioning system applied to trajectory analysis. American Roentgen Ray Society. April 2010.
8. Fischer T, Shogan P, Bunger R, Frew M, Provenzale J, Folio L. Anatomic positioning system applied to trajectory analysis in combat casualties. European Society of Radiologists; Vienna, Austria. May 2010.
9. Zhen J, Liu C, Wang S, Liu S, He J, Wang J, Chen H. The thin sectional anatomy of the temporal bone correlated with multislice spiral CT. Surg Radiol Anat. 2007 Jul; 29(5):409–18. (Epub 2007 Jun 22)
10. Backus C, Folio L. Lung laceration with active bleeding, contusion and hemothorax. Mil Med. 2008 Aug; 173(8):xv–xvi
11. Folio L, Fischer T. Backus C. Determining trajectories of ricocheting blast and ballistic fragments from complex wound paths. Mil Med. Pending date.
12. Willson T, Folio L. Severe epistaxis from an intracranial vascular bleed from grenade injury. Mil Med. 2008 Sept; 173(9):v–vi.
13. Fischer T, Folio L. Abdominal blast injury resulting in liver laceration, diaphragm disruption, hemothorax. Mil Med. Pending date.
14. Jackson AM, Searcey BK, Smirniotopoulos JG, Folio L. Keyhole fracture of the skull. Mil Med. 2008 Dec; 173(12):xix–xx.
15. Oehmichen M, Meissner C, Konig HG et al. Gunshot injuries to the head and brain caused by low-velocity handguns and rifles: a review. Forensic Sci Int. 2004; 146 (2–3):111–120.
16. Pabuscu Y, Bulakbasi N, Kocaoglu M et al. A different approach to missile induced head injuries. Comput Med Imaging Graph. 2003; 27 (5):397–409.
17. Di Maio VJ. Wounds from civilian and military centerfire rifles. Clin Lab Med. 1998 Jun; 18 (2):189–201.
18. Di Maio VJ, Spitz WU. Injury by birdshot. J Forensic Sci. 1970 Jul; 15(3):396–402.
19. Fischer T, Folio L. Abdominal blast injury resulting in liver laceration, diaphragmdisruption, hemothorax. Mil Med. 2011 Sept; 176(09).
20. Fischer T, Folio L. Abdominal blast injury resulting in liver laceration, diaphragm disruption, hemothorax. Mil Med. 2011 Sept; 176(09).
21. Fischer T, Folio L. Ricocheting blast injury fragment. Mil Med. 2011 Aug; 176(08):
22. Andrews C, Andrews K, Folio L. Venous fragment embolism to the pulmonary artery: a rare occurrence — case report and literature review of venous fragment embolization to the pulmonary artery. Mil Med. 2009 Sept; 174(9):iv,v.
23. Folio L, McHugh C, Hoffman MJ. The even-number guide and imaging ballistic injuries. Radiol Technol. 2007; 78:197–203.

24. Folio L, Robinson D. Apical hemothorax from gunshot wound producing a pleural cap. Mil Med. 2009 Dec; 174(12):vii–viii.
25. Folio L, Fischer T. Anatomic Positioning System: Blast and ballistic trajectory analysis using Multi-Detector Computerized Tomography (MD CT). American Society of Emergency Radiologists Annual Convention; Orlando, FL. 1 2009 Oct.
26. Gardocki RJ, Watkins RG, Williams LA. Measurements of lumbopelvic lordosis using the pelvic radius technique as it correlates with sagittal spinal balance and sacral translation. Spine J. 2002 Nov–Dec; 2(6):421–429.
27. Folio LR, Sears S, Lacy T. Teleradiology roundtable. Mil Med Technol. July 2007; 11(4): 6–11.
28. Folio L. Air force Telehealth Experience in Iraq. Diagnostic Imaging. 2005 Aug.
29. Folio L. Pak S. Patent Pending Serial Number: 11/447,516: G CROSS-SECTIONAL DIGITAL IMAGING INTO MOVIE FILE FORMAT. Filed in Patent and Trademark Office: 2006 June.
30. Folio L. Whitworth S. Universal Trauma Window Application in Damage Control Radiology. Exhibit/presentation at American Society of Emergency Radiology. 2009 Oct.
31. Shogan P, Folio L. A Standard, Secure and Universally Compatible Electronic Health Record for All Military, All Americans and Possibly All Nations by 2010. RSNA Exhibit. 2009.
32. Lodox Systems, North America, LLC. Available at: http://www.lodox.com (Accessed on Nov 24 2006).
33. Mirvis S. Use of total body digital radiography (Statscan) for acute trauma imaging: preliminary experience in comparison with traditional computed tomography. Available at: http:// rsna2005.rsna.org/rsna2005/V2005/conference/event_display.cfm?em_id=441427611

Chapter 6
Imaging Thresholds of Salvageability of Life, Limb, and Eyesight

Keywords Salvageability · Traumatic brain injury · Imaging mortality threshold · Radiology-assisted autopsy

6.1 Introduction

Important considerations in triage and re-triage are identifying the most critical casualties and separating out those who can be saved, and injuries so severe (expectant) that trying to save would unnecessarily drain resources from those who could live. The challenge of recent advances now saving more lives than ever is shifting the mortality threshold toward the more severe injuries; many considered expectant in prior conflicts and put to the side to die in the past are now saved. Perhaps, the most dramatic example of this is in head injuries with advent of faster transport times to neurosurgical capability on the battlefield as mentioned previously, and MDCT availability with correlations showing better survival predictability. Additionally, extremities not previously salvageable now are readily diagnosed by CTA (for example) with volume rendered 3D and multi-planar reformations with tools such as vessel tracking.

The most urgent situations anywhere in emergency management traditionally call for (and still call for), the saving of life, limb, and eyesight. In deployed combat hospitals in hostile territories, this mantra is what dictates what noncombat injuries and conditions of the local population will be treated at combat hospitals. Since the military capability often exceeds local country medical abilities, those too severe to be saved at local hospitals are transported to combat hospitals. Once saved with modern coalition forces technologies and capabilities, patients are transferred back to host nation medical care.

A paradoxical tradeoff of increased survival results in more living patients with more severe injuries than ever before. An example is the large number of soldiers, sailors, airman, and contracted civilians sent to war that are left with lost limbs; many times several limbs having been amputated. Fortunately, advances in prosthetic technologies have progressed to the point of helping these otherwise disabling wounds to be coped with better than ever before.

L. Folio (ed.), *Combat Radiology: Diagnostic Imaging of Blast and Ballistic Injuries*, DOI 10.1007/978-1-4419-5854-9_6, © Springer Science+Business Media, LLC 2010

Cases will be presented in this chapter on both sides of the current imaging life and death threshold to put this concept into perspective. Based on our experiences at the only combat hospital in Iraq with neurosurgical capability, imaging severity spectrums will be proposed that are still in need of further validation. I believe that standardizing the terminology and methods of consistent reporting from this point on will be imperative for epidemiological purposes and more effective data mining in the future when looking back at imaging findings and correlating with outcomes. A few extremity cases are also presented to demonstrate how CTA can guide surgeons to determine limb salvageability. The last section will present several penetrating globe injuries of various severity where some globes and vision were saved, others not so fortunate.

6.2 Pushing the Imaging Threshold of Mortality: Cases on the Edge of Life

6.2.1 Imaging Spectrum of Penetrating and Perforating Head Trauma on the Battlefield

Our hospital is the main hub for neurosurgical cases in Iraq. In addition, all HEENT related casualties in need of definitive treatment are seen at Balad Air Base. Of note, penetrating brain injuries from IEDs far much better than those with nearly identical scans that result from higher-energy projectiles (i.e., gunshot wounds) are seen in the US. Blast fragments can be high velocity, but are typically low-velocity and can cause less damage, even though fragments are often large. The CT results are compared with GCS score and used in concert with CT findings to fully evaluate prognosis.

Traditionally, Non Enhanced CT (NECT) was performed on mTBI (mild Traumatic Brain Injury). Based on evolving science and experience of our neurosurgical and diagnostic imaging teams, we considered to include CTP (CT Perfusion) imaging to provide the most sensitive baseline possible. Even though there is a paucity of prospective studies to prove that perfusion imaging is more sensitive in mTBI detection than CT without contrast [1], there is no gold standard yet for diagnosing mTBI definitively (MRI is not a possibility in deployed combat hospitals at the time of this writing). Until then, we considered using the most sensitive tool possible in a combat environment. There are several neurocognitive tests depending on the level of facility and workup. Front-line screening on suspected mTBI is performed with the Military Acute Concussion Evaluation (MACE). Theater referral center evaluation involves Automated Neuropsychological Assessment Metrics (ANAM).

"No head injury is too trivial to ignore" (Hippocrates, 460–377 BC, in Ingebrigsten) [2]

Missile injuries and CT severity have been addressed in the literature with Shoung et al. reporting on 56 cases and correlating to CT [3] and Kaufman et al. describing two cases where aggressive treatment allowed salvage in cases previously thought not to be possible [4].

There are many recent advances in TBI, to include extensive craniotomy techniques with more severe head injuries. At the onset of the recent campaign in Iraq, a skull flap was removed and placed into the abdomen for later recovery [5]. This was soon replaced by computer-aided design and manufacturing of methomethacralate synthetic implants mirrored from the normal half of the skull for optimal cosmetic fit.

In our experience in the only combat hospital in Iraq with neurosurgical capability, the image severity findings of penetrating trauma on CT exhibited a predictable parallel clinical prognosis spectrum. In other words, neurosurgeons and radiologists could come to conclusions quickly as to prognosis of survivability when it came to CT triage (expectant vs. survivable severe injury).

While deployed, I developed a standard report to allow radiologists to more effectively communicate penetrating head injury findings to neurosurgeons, emergency department physicians, and ICU medical staff. The written preliminary triage report was easier for radiologists to complete in that parameters could be circled with a yes or no rather than writing out each time (most everyone preferred the binary yes / no circles over my handwriting). Medical staff could quickly assess the findings important to them. Prior to this, neurosurgeons had to search for information buried in a nonstandard report in various orders depending on each of the radiologist's style. Standardized reporting of penetrating head injuries provided more efficient communication to neurosurgeons and other hospital medical staff over several months.

Parameters on the standard report include presence or absence of the following: Pneumocephalus, missile path (bihemispheric, multilobar, transventricular), skull fracture, evidence of elevated intracranial pressure (effaced sulci, basal cisterns, midline shift, etc.), hemorrhage (location choices: cisternal, SAH, IVH, extraaxial), and intraparenchymal hemorrhage. These parameters were arranged in a consistent table format with checklist-type responses (see Fig. 6.1). In addition to saving radiologist time, ED docs, trauma surgeons, neurosurgeons, orthopedic surgeons, etc. knew instantly where to look for the findings of their interest. Figure 6.2 is a zoomed up view of the head CT standard section. This minimized writing (a good thing in my case), and again, standardized our reporting in the parameters that radiologists and neurosurgeons found important. By completing this form that also acted as a checklist, told the neurosurgeon the questions they would have before arriving to include pertinent negatives (rather than going back and asking about pneumocephalus for example).

These preliminary reports were later entered into each casualty's computer medical record that would go with them through the medical echelons back to their home medical centers. The consistent format made it easier for the radiologist to look back on what was reported for entering into our EHR.

Another advantage to the standard reporting is consistent data mining in the future. Since we were seeing more penetrating head trauma than ever before, with

Radiology Form: Trauma/ Surge/ MassCal

332 EMDG   AGE:____   US Name, trauma # or TCN/LN #

Radiology Phone 443-8527   NOTE: for mass casualty, can substitute Trauma Number only for Name and SSN

Rad Tech Name: **Time of Exam:**   SS#   -   -

Location: ER 443-8513					**Date:** Day Month Year
From:	Field	10th	FOB:	Other:	

History: (Circle one)   IED   Mortar   Gunshot   MVA   EET   Central Line   NG/OG Tube

Provider/ER staff: Please circle requested exams:

X-Ray Exams			Results
CXR		CXR by CT Scout	
		Pelvis	
Other (eg. KUB, Lat C Spine)			
RT	LT	SHOULDER	
RT	LT	HUMERUS	
RT	LT	ELBOW	
RT	LT	FOREARM	
RT	LT	WRIST	
RT	LT	HAND	
RT	LT	FEMUR	
RT	LT	KNEE	
RT	LT	TIB/FIB	
RT	LT	ANKLE	
RT	LT	FOOT	

CT Exams

PanScan	Head	Negative	Positive (if positive, fill out below findings)

Head section (Positive findings):

Missile track? No Yes	Unilobar?: No Yes (___ lobe)	Bihemispheric? No Yes	Multilobar? No Yes	Transventricular? No Yes
CT findings c/w elevated ICP? No Yes		Sulci? Effaced Patent	Cisterns? Patent Effaced	Midline shift? No Yes (_____ mm)
Hemorrhage? No Yes	Intraparenchymal hemorrhage? No Yes ___x___x___mm ___lobe		Cisternal? SAH? IVH?	Extra-axial? No Yes (_DH)
Pneumocephalus? No Yes			Other:	

		Results
	C-Spine	
	Chest	
	Abdomen	
	Pelvis	
	CTA COW	
	CT Face	
	CTA Carotids	
	CTA Chest	
	Other (eg. T+L Spine)	

Findings Continued on Back if Checked ☐

Additional forms available on t drive under T:\Radiology\Admin Files\Forms

Updated 21 July 2007

FIRMR (41 CRF) 101-11.806-8

Fig. 6.1 I designed this handwritten report (modified from prior versions) while we were deployed to allow quick ordering of imaging studies in a consistent fashion while standardizing where results were reported by radiologists on the sheet. This was easier for radiologists in that there was less writing, at the same time medical staff knew where to look for the results they were interested in for more efficient communications

	CT Exams				
	Negative	Positive (if positive, fill out below findings)			
Head	**Missile track?** No Yes	**Unilobar?:** No Yes (___ lobe)	**Bihemispheric?** No Yes	**Multilobar?** No Yes	**Transventricular?** No Yes
	CT findings c/w elevated ICP? No		**Sulci?** Effaced Patent	**Cisterns?** Patent	**Midline shift?** No Yes (______ mm)
	Hemorrhage? No Yes		**Intraparenchymal ?** No Yes ___ x ___ x ___ mm ___ lobe	Cisternal? SAH? IVH?	**Extra-axial?** No Yes (_DH)
	Pneumocephalus? No Yes	Other:			
C-Spine					
Chest					
Abdomen					
Pelvis					

Fig. 6.2 Section of the standard report that provided the information radiologists would place findings and that neurosurgeons agreed was the key information important to them. This was also helpful to nursing staff that had certain parameters to look for in follow-up care

some severe casualties surviving that had not survived previously, we felt it was important to capture this information in a way easier to correlate with clinical notes down the road.

The Marshall grading scale [6–9] was kept into consideration when developing this format with our neurosurgery department. When data from our Electronic Medical Record (EMR) is later accessed for evidence-based treatment and studies, this data can be consistently mined. This also simplifies where to look for the result and allows consistency in reporting with constantly changing radiologists. The ICU and neurosurgical teams can know that everything dealing with penetrating trauma was reviewed. Since the reports are handwritten initially (later entered into our EMR, JPTA), this minimizes extra writing and simplifies data entry.

Survivability surrogates, or CT grading of penetrating trauma, may be able to be determined after review of consistent data. Although a "CT GCS" is not proposed here, perhaps this is not an impossible concept in the future, based on clinical record review, CT findings (organized as above), and mechanism of injury. Once we become more familiar with penetrating head injury to include blast, resource (time, blood, staff, OR) determination may be better estimated by determining nonsurvivable (expectant) versus. survivable CT findings.

The real-estate mantra holds true, especially in penetrating and perforating injuries to the brain: location, location, location. I like to break each of these locations into their own category. Location #1: Entrance, Location #2: Exit (or resultant missile remnant), and Location #3: Trajectory: wound ballistics. One needs to ask, "what path did the missile take (hence, what organs were involved)?" in that the trajectory real-estate should be considered, not just the entrance and final location (or exit).

A severity scale based on these consistent findings was proposed in a case review of several traumatic brain injury cases [10]. The authors showed several cases of closed head injury of increasing severity to include a negative CT and MR, negative CT and positive MR (only on GRE), and positive CT and positive MR. Some authors have reviewed trajectories of GSW and related to outcomes [11]. A severity scale is being further studied at USU [12]. Penetrating head trauma CT studies are being reviewed and correlated with example reports, using the report format discussed above. The CT report format is being compared to neurosurgical procedures and findings with other predictability measures to include GCS and clinical follow-up of patients. Computer modeling may be applied to help determine survivability. Quantification and prognosis scores similar to Glasgow Coma Scale (GCS) and Injury Severity Score (ISS) may be possible with similar standard formats used over time. There is a paucity of literature on accuracy of trajectory measurements and actual locations in the brain, and especially the body.

6.3 Example Penetrating Head Injury Cases in Increasing Severity

A child fell head-first onto an 8″ long pipe (about 1″ in diameter) sticking in the ground. Since it happened in a remote area of Iraq without communication capability, the father pulled the child from the pipe and brought to our combat hospital. Since this is qualified as a life or death situation, even though the child was alert, crying, no reported LOC, with GCS 13, and stable vital signs, the pipe penetrated deep enough to effect the child's vision. A deep laceration was noted superior and right of the frontal sinus. A CT was performed and seen in the following Figures (Figs. 6.3–6.10).

While these images seem to indicate a severe penetrating head injury case, because of the brain area involved, the quick neurosurgical intervention and release of pressure and the mechanism, this child was not only saved, he was discharged after a few days on antibiotics.

For an intermediate perforating head injury case, refer to the keyhole injury discussed in the previous chapter. This case highlights a focused entrance and exit with indriven bone fragments that is often fatal. Due to immediate neurosurgical intervention, this casualty was saved as the keyhole pattern was recognized to be a serious injury even though it could initially seem trivial.

The following unfortunate case shows a perforating head injury case from a suicide. Figure 6.11 shows the entrance in the right parietal region of this right-handed soldier's head, with large open fracture and fragments. The bullet direction is shown by the arrow and traverses the midline and ventricles, a grave indicator. Note the blood in the ventricles, swelling, and midline shift. Figure 6.12 shows the exit on a higher cut. This person lived long enough to get the scans; however, with a GCS of three and other clinical indicators of death, this was not a salvageable injury. This upward right to left angle is consistent with a right-handed, close range, self-inflicted incident. Left-handed individuals would have a mirror image pattern and also inferior to superior.

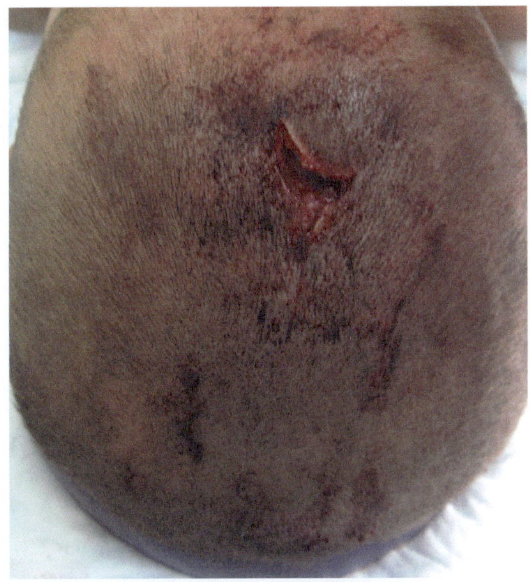

Fig. 6.3 Photo of child's head from the top just prior to neurosurgery showing the skin laceration from the pipe injury. Reprinted with permission from Military Medicine: International Journal of AMSUS

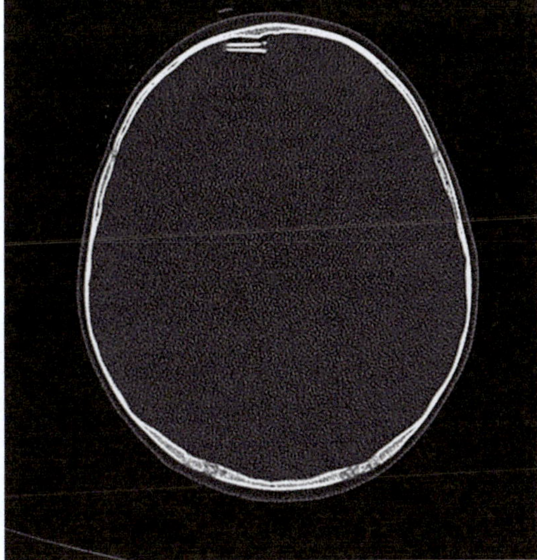

Fig. 6.4 Axial NCCT bone windows demonstrating a perplexing bone flap inside the right frontal bone. Reprinted with permission from Military Medicine: International Journal of AMSUS

6.4 Blast and Ballistic Injuries to the Neck

Penetrating neck injuries are a common cause of death in combat in that the body armor does not always cover the neck region major vasculature and airway. Penetrating trauma to the carotids results in extravasation or pseudoaneurysm as seen in the case in the previous chapter. That patient was saved due to severity of

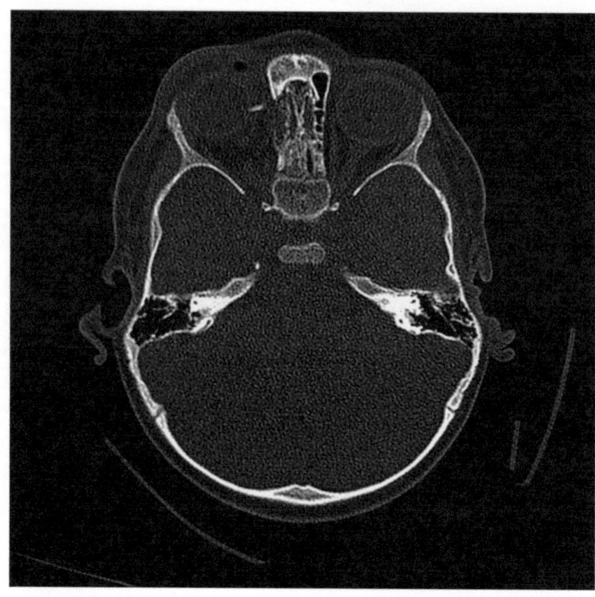

Fig. 6.5 Another axial bone window view now showing a bone fragment medial to the right orbit presumably from the nearby fractured lamina papyracea. Note the orbital emphysema as well. Reprinted with permission from Military Medicine: International Journal of AMSUS

Fig. 6.6 A coronal bone window again showing the bone flap in the extra-axial space in the right frontal region. Reprinted with permission from Military Medicine: International Journal of AMSUS

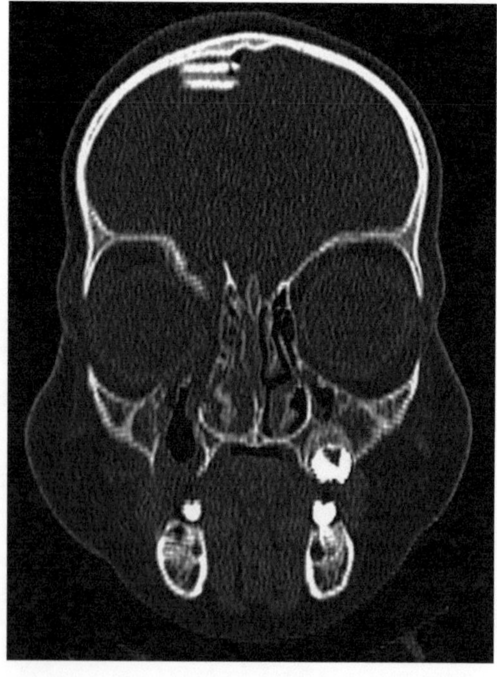

Fig. 6.7 Another coronal now helping explain the pipe entrance and how the pipe penetrated the skull. Reprinted with permission from Military Medicine: International Journal of AMSUS

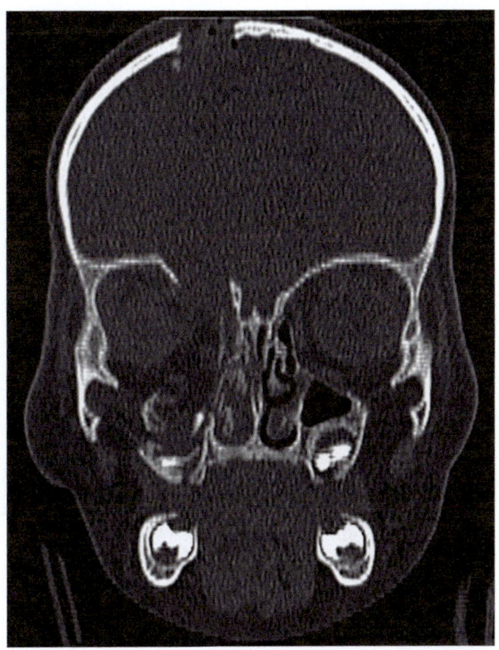

Fig. 6.8 The same coronal view now with an animated pipe showing what the neurosurgeon and I felt had happened based on the imaging and neurosurgical findings. Reprinted with permission from Military Medicine: International Journal of AMSUS

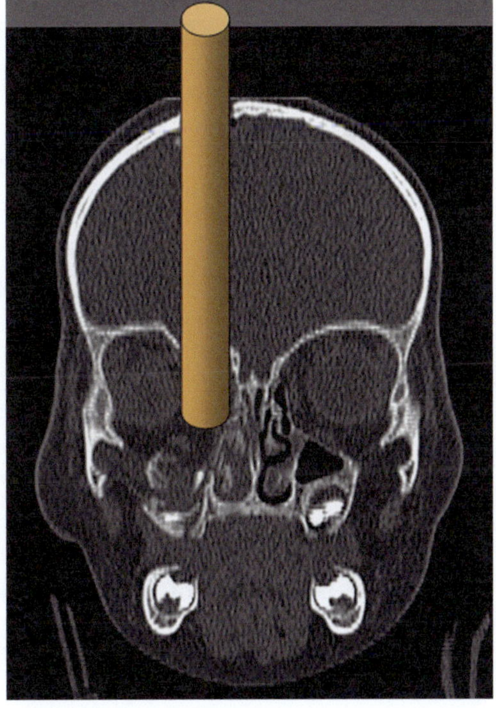

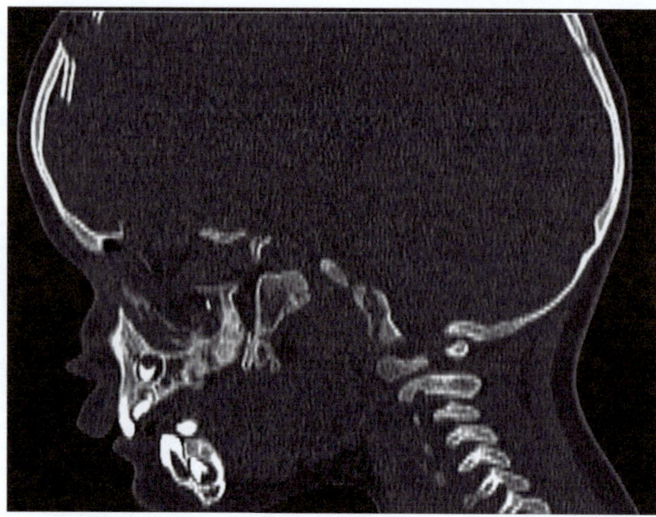

Fig. 6.9 A sagittal bone window CT reformat further explaining the skull flap that had essentially flipped under the skull from the pipe penetration. Also note damage to the orbital floor in the width of the pipe. Reprinted with permission from Military Medicine: International Journal of AMSUS

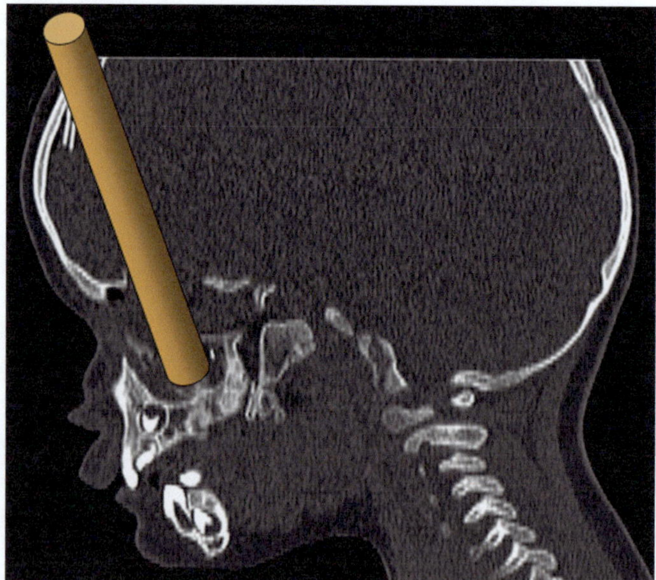

Fig. 6.10 The same sagittal CT reformat from above, now with the animated pipe to demonstrate the severity of the injury. Reprinted with permission from Military Medicine: International Journal of AMSUS

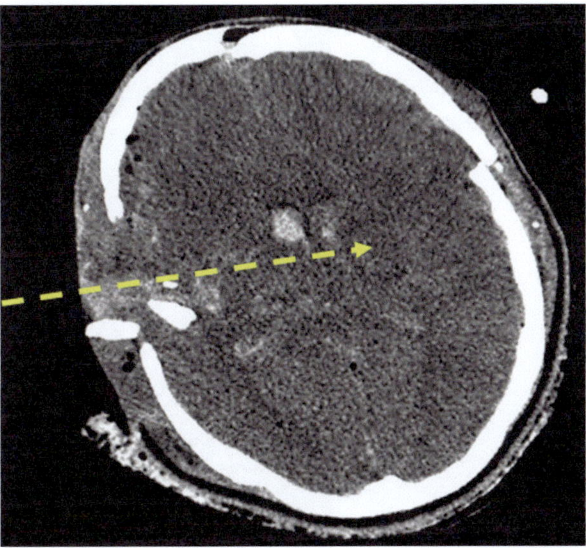

Fig. 6.11 Note the entrance of this patient that committed suicide. Note the angle of the bullet that crossed the midline, also blood in the lateral ventricles anteriorly, swelling of brain, loss of gray-white matter differentiation, pneumocephalus, indriven bone fragments. Reprinted with permission from Military Medicine: International Journal of AMSUS

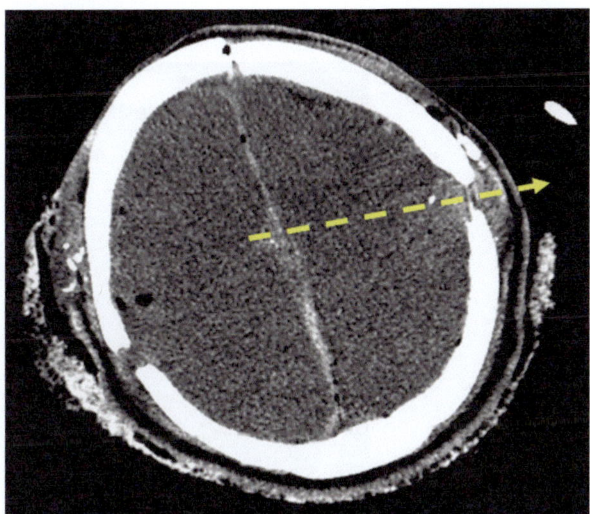

Fig. 6.12 The exit wound was higher and exhibited beveling to support this and clinical indicators of exit. Close range shots like this will have a reversal of the exit and entrance wound size expectations in that the exit is sometimes smaller than the entrance. Reprinted with permission from Military Medicine: International Journal of AMSUS

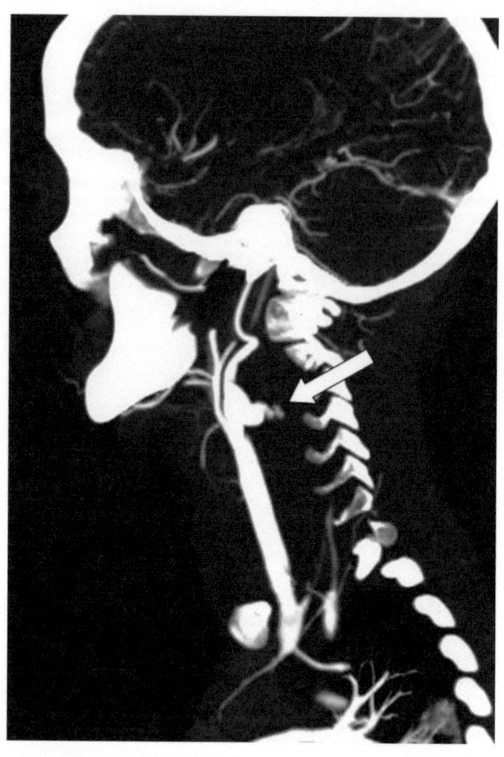

Fig. 6.13 Child caught in firefight shot in the neck with resultant pseudoaneurysm on CTA (*arrow*)

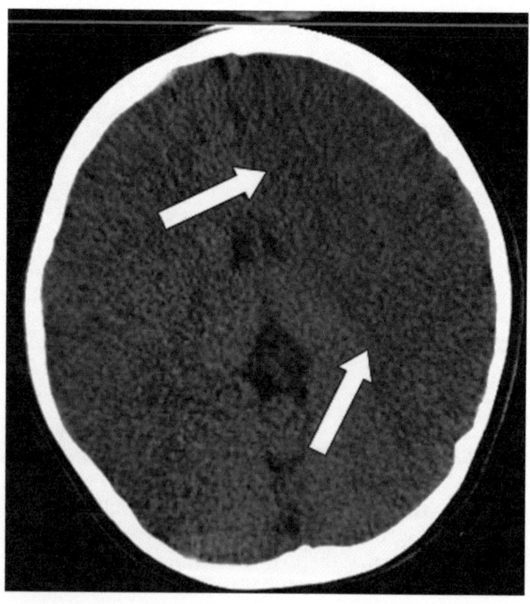

Fig. 6.14 Noncontrast CT showing large ACA, MCA distribution infarct (*arrows*)

injury and rapid evacuation to neurointerventional capability. Another case of a pseudoaneurysm in a child, however, was not so fortunate. See Fig. 6.13 for the CTA MIP of the carotids of a 7 year old shot through the neck accidently in a firefight. Note the large pseudoaneurysm on the left that resulted in severe neck distension. This was not a survivable injury, however, due to presumed clots from the carotid injury on the left. See CT of head without contrast for large ACA, MCA infarct (Fig. 6.14).

The previous chapter showed a GSW to the neck in a soldier that lived only long enough to survive the trip to the hospital. This bullet went through the spinal cord in the cervical spine region high enough to deem the patient insalvageable.

6.5 Eyesight Salvageability in Penetrating Trauma

Despite aggressive preventive measures with eye protection and education, a significant number of ocular injuries have occurred during recent combat operations mostly due to blast injuries. Many include intraocular foreign bodies from IED fragmentation. Advances in ophthalmologic microsurgery have significantly incre-ased the chances of globe salvageability. Also, the use of computed tomography in theater has been instrumental in showing the extent of injury. Several cases of orbital trauma are reviewed here with analysis of each injury seen on CT scan. A discussion follows as to whether the globe in each case was salvageable. More information on these and other cases have been described and will be published soon [13].

Several factors have been identified as to globe salvage probability in penetrating trauma. Factors that usually lead to a good prognosis include an anterior wound location, wounds less than 10 mm in size, initial visual acuity at the time of injury to be 20/200 or greater, and a sharp intraocular foreign body(causes less ocular disruption) [14]. CT has only recently been considered in determining salvageability, however, may add to the prognosis equation significantly.

Lemeley et al. [15] lists several factors associated with globe loss after an intraocular foreign body injury. Poor prognostic factors included a wound larger than 10 mm, injuries that involved the retina, an afferent papillary defect, initial visual acuity less than 5/200 at the time of injury, and injuries from blunt objects (such as BBs).

Ehlers et al. [16] found similar prognostic factors when they analyzed 96 patients with metallic foreign body injuries. The factors most strongly associated with globe loss were an afferent papillary defect, BB/pellet mechanism of injury, and no light perception at the time of injury. Excellent visual outcome (>20/50) after injury was associated with a normal lens at presentation, an anterior segment IOFB, and vision better than 20/200 at time of presentation. Organic foreign bodies also tend to have a worse prognosis because they are more prone to infection or inflammatory reaction [17].

Computed Tomography was used as the primary imaging modality when these patients were first evaluated in the combat causality hospital. CT provides invaluable information when evaluating penetrating orbital injuries. It provides the location of any foreign bodies, visualization of soft tissues, and determination of whether the globe has been ruptured or perforated. It can also demonstrate whether the injury is isolated to the orbit or if there is associated intracranial and paranasal sinus injury. Computed tomography can help determine the extent of injury and identify those factors that are associated with globe salvageability and globe loss.

MRI and Ultrasound are additional imaging modalities that can be used to assess intraocular foreign bodies. These imaging modalities, however, were not used in the combat hospital due to limited resources and space. MRI does provide better resolution if the IOFB is made of organic material. MRI may also give better resolution for detecting optic nerve lacerations or optic nerve avulsions [18]. However, caution must be used before using MRI as it potentially could cause further injury if the foreign body is ferromagnetic. Ultrasound can also assist in detecting both radiolucent and radio-dense intraocular foreign bodies to provide more information on size, shape, and relative position.

See Fig. 6.15 for an axial image of a face CT, which shows a blast fragment that penetrated deep into the right orbit. While only one fragment is seen in this image, several fragments were seen retrobulbar after CT analysis. Only one fragment tangentially affected the globe (Fig. 6.16). The right eye was salvaged in this case. The important factor in this case was that while several fragments did penetrate the orbit, none of the fragments penetrated the globe.

This axial image of a head CT shows several metallic fragments located in the left globe (Fig. 6.17). There is also a small left-sided temporal lobe hematoma. In this case, the metallic fragments have penetrated the left globe. While the globe has

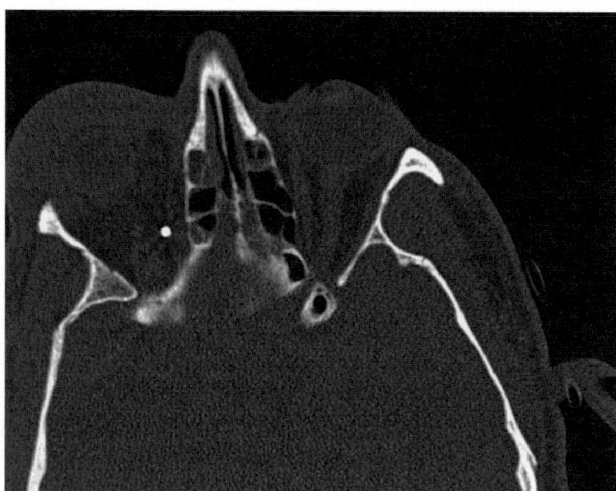

Fig. 6.15 Axial image of face CT show metal fragment in the right orbit with no compromise to the globe. Note severe soft tissue swelling anterior to the right globe. Reprinted with permission from Military Medicine: International Journal of AMSUS

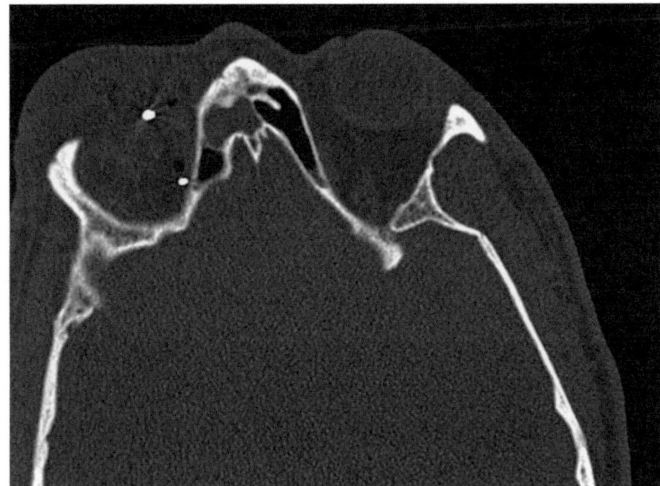

Fig. 6.16 Axial image of face CT demonstrating metal fragment tangentially effecting right globe with minimal disturbance to globe integrity. Globe and eyesight were salvaged in this case

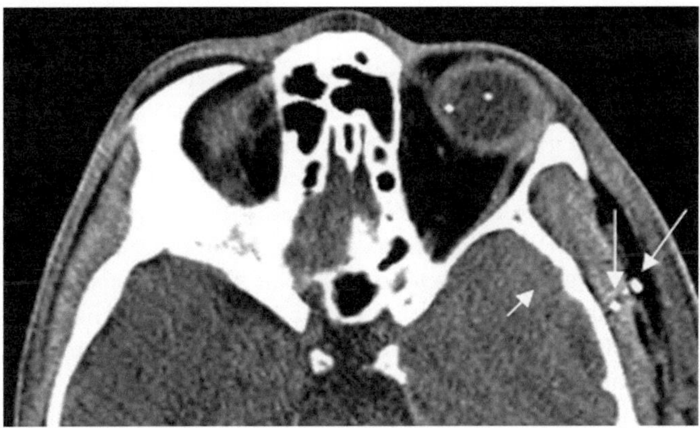

Fig. 6.17 Axial image of head CT shows two metallic fragments in the left globe. This globe was salvageable. Note the small left temporal lobe bleed (*short arrow*) and two other blast fragments and sub-q air on the left superficial facial soft tissues (*long arrows*). The right globe was not involved and not seen on this slice due to partial volume. Reprinted with permission from Military Medicine: International Journal of AMSUS

been penetrated, the globe integrity is still maintained. The total number of fragments are relatively few with just two penetrating the globe. The globe in this case was salvageable, and this was largely due to the ability to close the globe soon after injury. The small size of the metallic fragments and relatively few number of fragments in this globe also were factors in globe salvageability.

Next case shows an axial image of a head/neck CTA that shows multiple metal fragments in the left and right orbit (Fig. 6.18). The right orbit was more severely

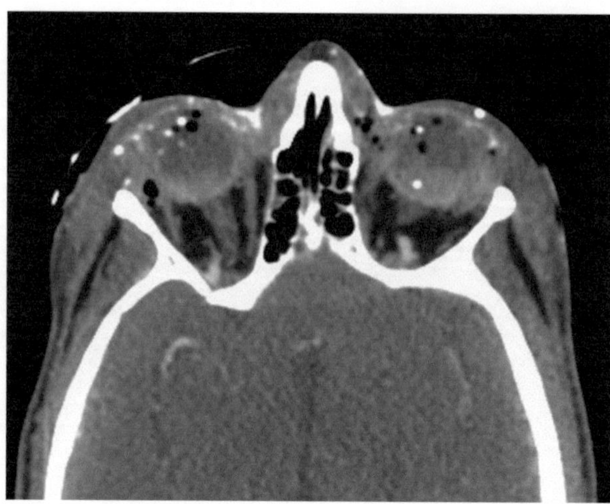

Fig. 6.18 CT image of orbits in shows multiple fragments within the right globe and left globe. These globes were not salvageable. Reprinted with permission from Military Medicine: International Journal of AMSUS

injured with significant fragmentation, eleven discrete areas of cavitation, and approximately 10% of air in the right globe. An attempt was made to salvage the right globe and the left globe. Unfortunately, the damage was too extensive in both globes to salvage due to the significant fragmentation.

The next case shows axial images of a head CT with two large fragments in the right globe (Figs. 6.19–6.21). The two fragments were removed in theater. The laceration to the right globe was extensive. Repair was attempted in theater, but the posterior aspect of the laceration could not be closed. Approximately, 20% of air was left in the globe after removal of the two fragments. When this patient was aero-evacuated, cabin altitude restrictions were required due to concerns of air expansion within the globe at altitude. Despite early intervention, this globe was not salvageable due to the size of fragmentation.

This is a sagital image of a head CT that shows a glass fragment penetrating the left globe (Fig. 6.22) from a blast. The glass fragment pierced the entire globe, and the damage was too extensive to salvage the eye. See Fig. 6.23 for operative photo of removed globe and glass.

CT shows bilateral globe disruptions from a gunshot wound crossing both eyes. This unfortunate casualty will never see again as both globes were immediately destroyed by a bullet crossing both eyes (Figs. 6.24–6.27).

Management of orbital trauma in a combat hospital offers many challenges but the primary goals are the same: immediate stabilization with closure of the globe and antibiotic administration. Definitive care may not occur until the patient is aeromedically evacuated out of theater. If there is significant air in the globe, consideration must be given to cabin altitude restrictions in the aircraft. A large

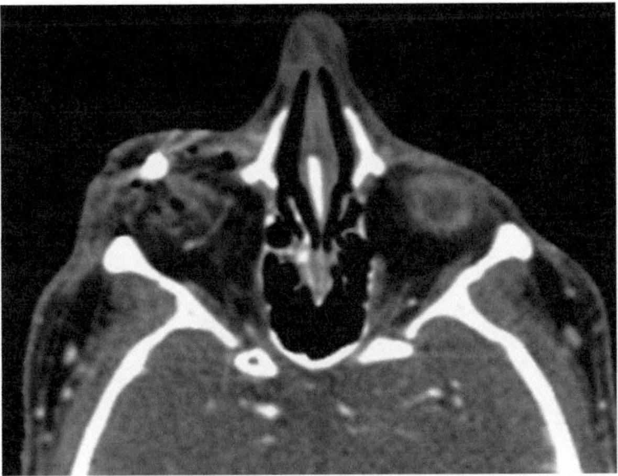

Fig. 6.19 CT axial image shows a large fragment lateral and anterior aspect of right globe with partially intruded right globe

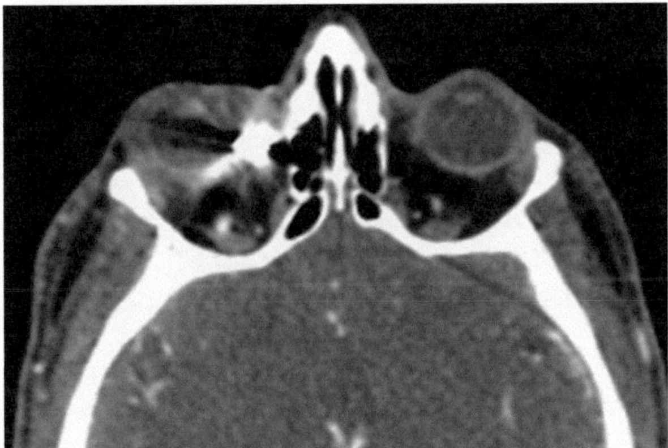

Fig. 6.20 CT axial slightly superior showing other large metallic fragment, this one in the medial aspect of globe

amount of air in the globe will expand at altitude (generally volume will double in size) and may cause further injury. Thus, cabin altitude restrictions may be required.

Removal of the foreign body may be delayed until after the patient has been evacuated, especially if the IOFB is posteriorly located and difficult to remove. There is some debate on whether delayed removal of an IOFB affects vision prognosis. Lemley et al. [19] found that a delay of 24 h in primary repair/removal of the foreign body increased the risk of endopthalmitis/severe vision loss fourfold. He goes on to state that delayed IOFB removal increases the formation of inflammatory fibrous tissue, condensation of the vitreous, and increases the risk of retinal

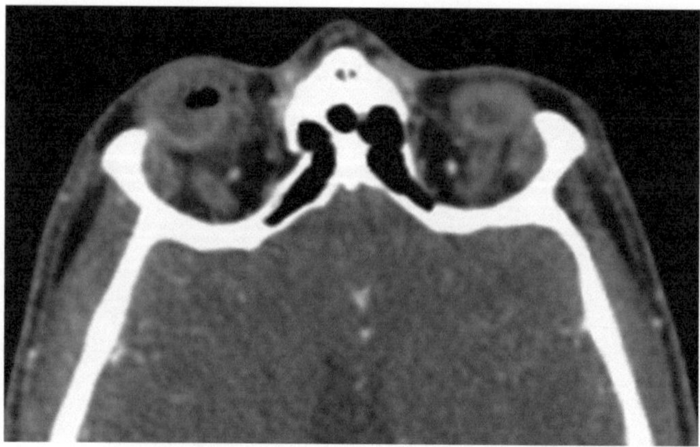

Fig. 6.21 More superior axial image showing significant air in right globe. It is important to quantify the amount of air within the globe to the flight surgeon before transport by aircraft

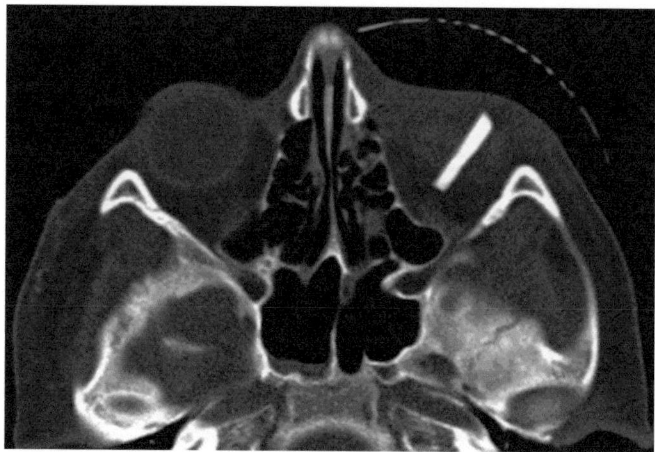

Fig. 6.22 CT axial bone window showing glass fragment that penetrated the left globe

detachment. However, recent studies of injured patients in Iraq have found that a delay in IOFB removal may not be as concerning as previously thought [20,21]. Ehlers et al. [22] in his own study found no significant association between time to surgical intervention and outcome. He goes on to say, "emergent IOFB removal may not be as necessary as previously thought as long as open-globe injury is closed promptly and systemic antibiotics are initiated quickly." The risk of endoopthalmitis after an open-globe injury was found to be 4–6% [23]. The risk of sympathetic opthalmia, a devastating complication of an open-globe injury, which results in vision loss of the uninjured eye has been low at 0.3% in recent studies [24].

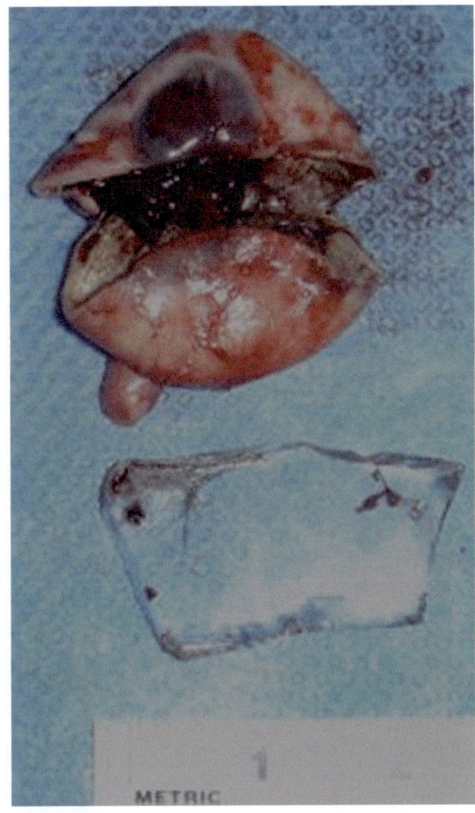

Fig. 6.23 Intraoperative photo of globe after removal with glass fragment that penetrated the left globe

If the globe is damaged beyond repair, evisceration is preferred over enucleation. Evisceration is technically easier and yields better cosmetic and functional results. In addition, enucleation can lead to several complications like hypoopthalmia, superior sulcus deformities, and motility disturbances [18]. These complications are minimized in eviscerations. Sympathetic opthalmia can occur but is generally very rare after evisceration [18].

These cases help illustrate the vast spectrum of ocular injuries that can occur after blasts. Computed Tomography can help to determine the extent of ocular injury. With more research in this area, CT grading may be possible in the future, providing further guidance on the extent of injury.

6.6 Imaging in Limb Salvage

Plain radiography, CT, CTA, and C-arm angiography can help orthopedic surgeons determine salvageability on the battlefield and what resources should be spent on surgical techniques such as vascular repair and external fixators. A few cases are

Fig. 6.24 Coronal image showing GSW path across both globes

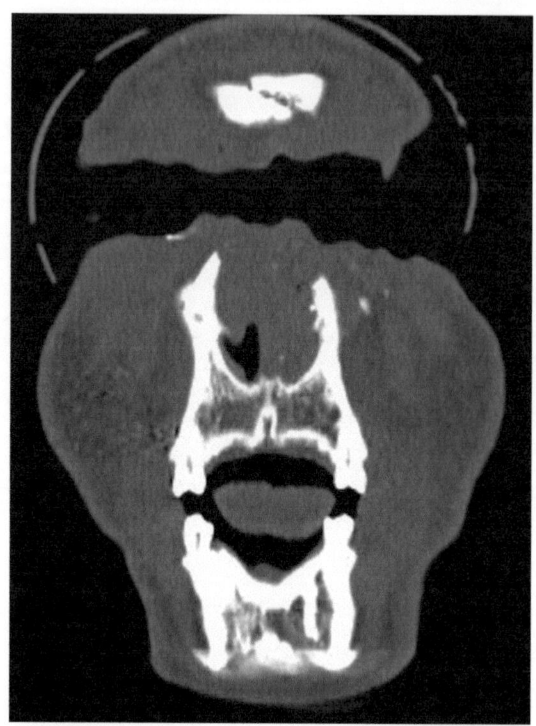

Fig. 6.25 Coronal image bone windows showing extensive facial fractures including frontal and maxillary sinuses

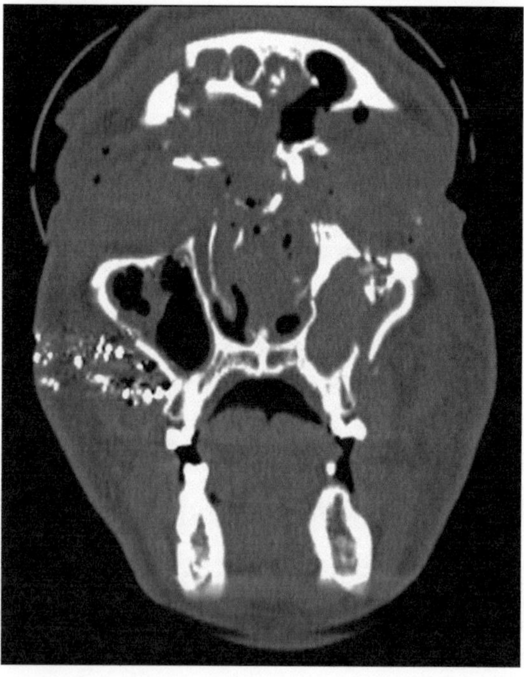

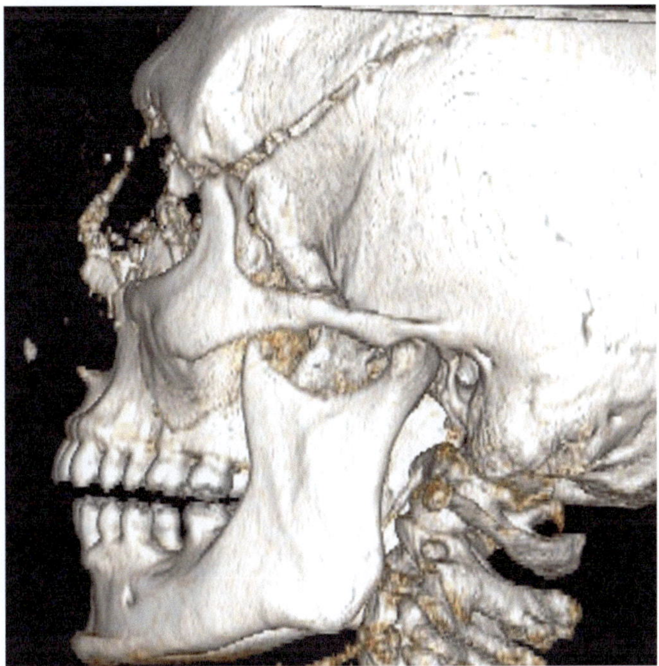

Fig. 6.26 Three dimensional volume rendered image looking through the bullet path just posterior to the nasal bones

presented to highlight how imaging can help guide trauma surgeons in saving extremities, where before CT were often not salvageable.

The first two cases highlight how CTA can quickly evaluate vascular status to the upper extremities. The first casualty was shot in the chest superiorly and centrally, with bullet transitioning through brachial region on left. A CTA of the chest was ordered to evaluate major vascular bleed. See Fig. 6.28 for the CT scout CXR showing the bullet, subcutaneous emphysema in the wound path, and a large hemothorax on the left. The bullet ended up posterior to the left scapula near the skin (Figs. 6.29–6.31).

The other case highlighting how CTA can help evaluate vessel integrity to an extremity is another GSW to the chest medial to lateral, going through the right scapula. See Fig. 6.32 for 3D rendered CT showing an intact left subclavian artery, in the path of a bullet that perforated the right scapula (Fig. 6.33).

This next case shows how a lower extremity CTA of a GSW to the thigh demonstrated a major extremity vascular injury. See Fig. 6.34 for a vessel tracking reformation of a CTA of the lower extremities. This thrombus in the femoral artery was repaired and resulted in saving of the leg based on CT localization.

Fig. 6.27 Photo from the side of this patient showing the wound path behind anterior superior nose

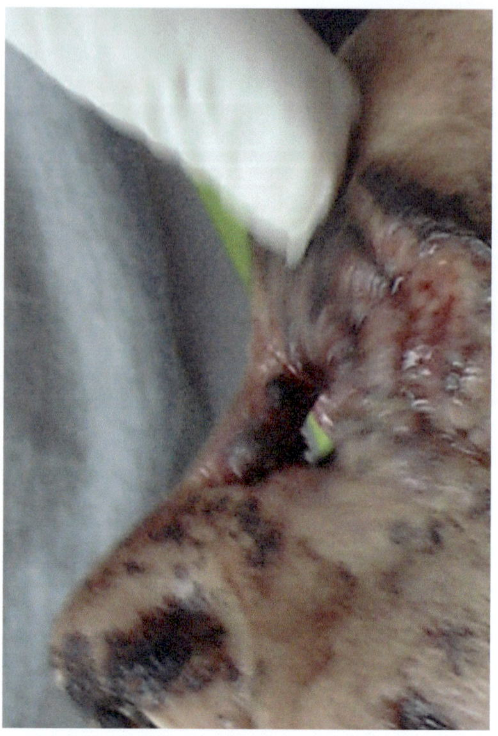

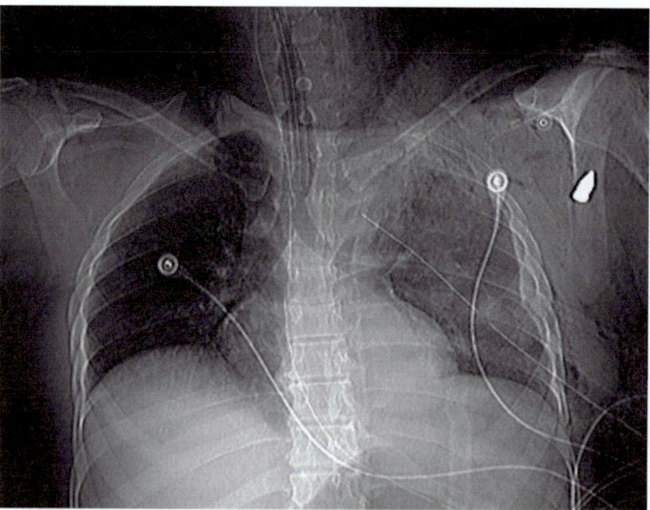

Fig. 6.28 CT scout CXR of casualty with GSW to the chest superiorly and left with weak pulse in left arm. Note large left hemothorax (especially toward apex) with subcutaneous emphysema in left axilla

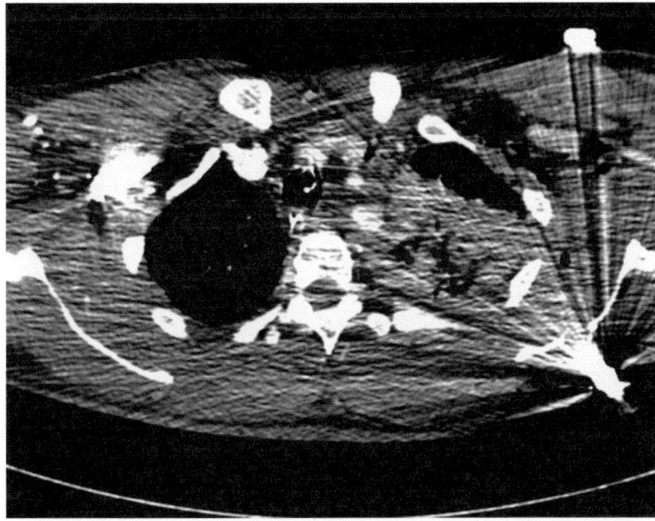

Fig. 6.29 CT Angiogram with bullet and lung contusion supporting anterior to posterior and medial to lateral wound path. Note great vessels partially seen (limited due to motion and, beam hardening)

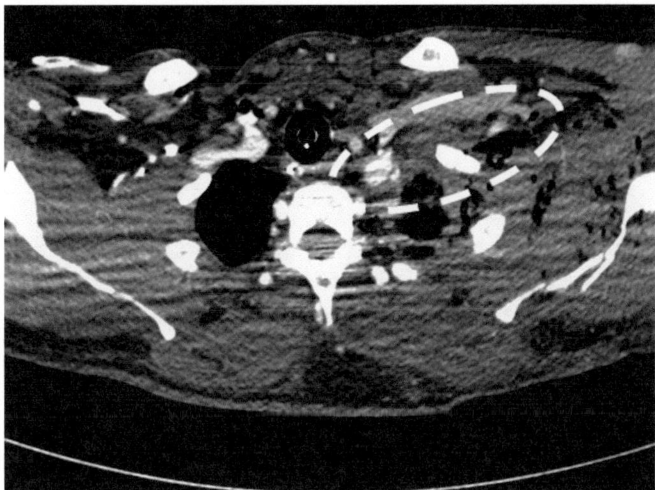

Fig. 6.30 CT Angiogram showing large subclavian artery disruption. This is better demonstrated on vessel tracking

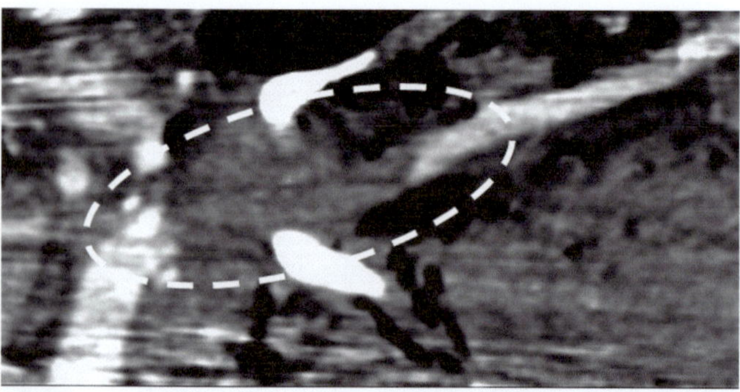

Fig. 6.31 CT vessel tracking reformat through left subclavian artery. This thrombus was repaired in surgery and the arm was salvaged

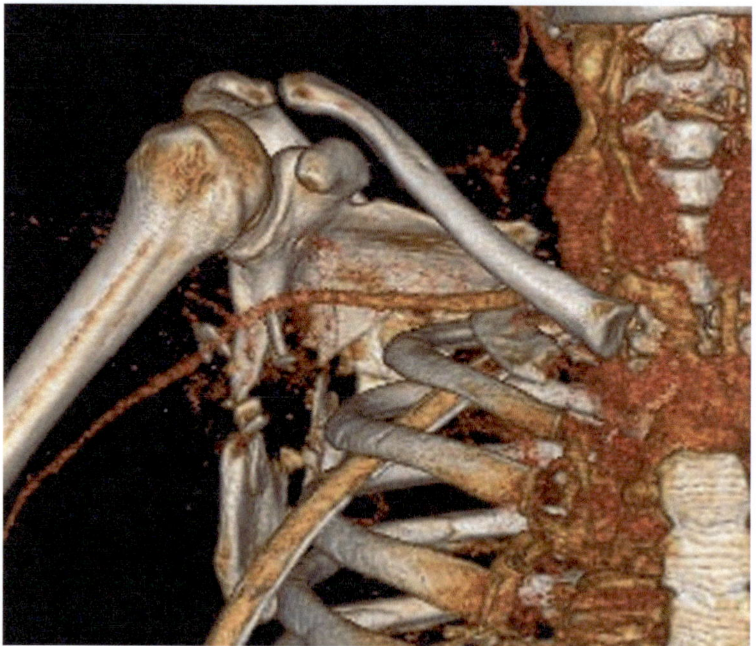

Fig. 6.32 Three dimensional CTA showing intact right subclavian that was in path of bullet that also perforated the right scapula

6.7   Radiology-Assisted Autopsy

An extensive review of forensic analysis is beyond the scope of this book, however, one should see from this chapter how imaging can play a pivotal role in cause of death, and more importantly, determining cause of life from an epidemiological

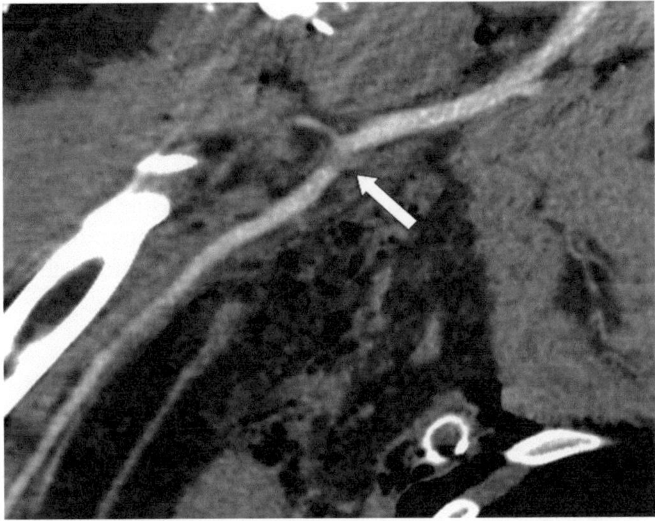

Fig. 6.33 CT vessel tracking showing the intact vessel. This image also shows how processing errors can be mistaken of thrombus (*arrow*)

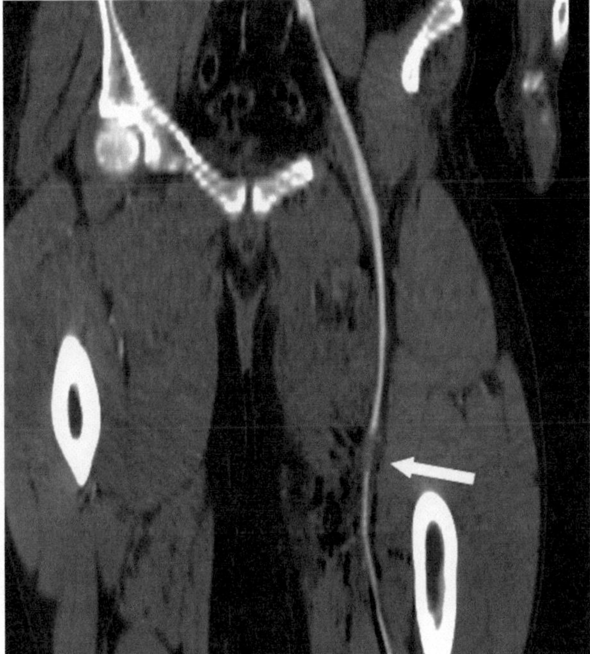

Fig. 6.34 CT vessel tracking of the left lower leg showing a large thrombus in the femoral artery in the region of the GSW path in the medial thigh. Note extensive subcutaneous emphysema medial to the vessel

perspective. By studying casualties that have lived from combat medicine in recent years that otherwise died in previous conflicts, we can see the impact imaging has made and where to continue to make improvements in combat casualty care. See Fig. 6.35 for a threshold graph I put together to show in presentations when discussing this topic. I believe that identifying the imaging mortality threshold of life, limb, and eyesight will help save more lives by changing perceptions of survival – potentially moving the threshold toward increasing survival in the future. Radiologists can not only help forensic pathologists determine the cause and manner of death, we can all help determine the cause of life in those that in the past would have died.

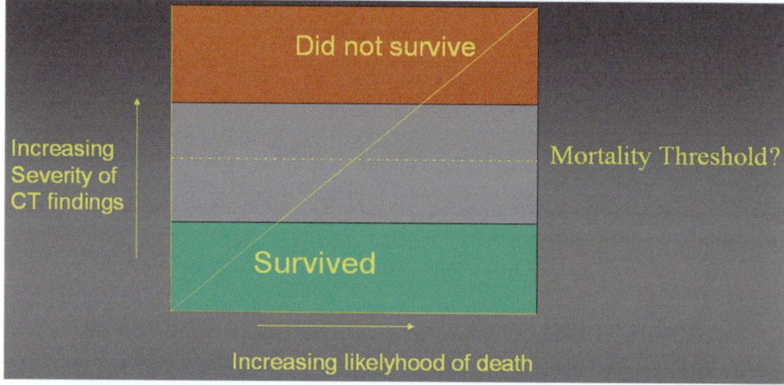

Fig. 6.35 A basic graph I show in presentations reflecting my perception on increasing severity of imaging findings and the resultant increasing likelihood of death based on worse imaging findings. I think most radiologists agree that there are findings so severe that death is imminent, especially true with head CT

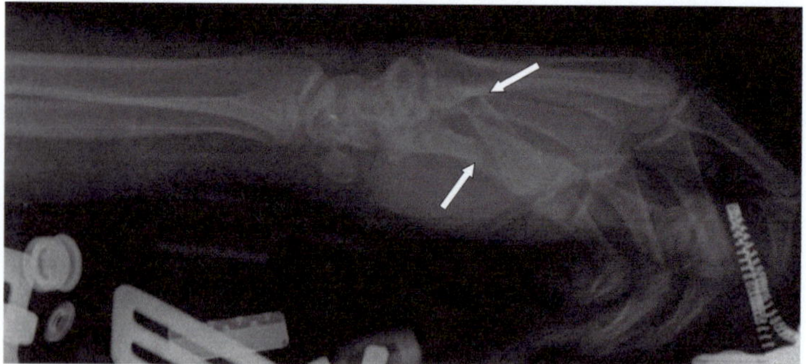

Fig. 6.36 Cyclic control injury: Plain X-ray of right hand of the flying pilot shows a posteriorly displaced transverse fracture of the fifth MC likely from contact with the cyclic rest on impact (*arrows* in e). There is also a subtle lucency through the base of the first MC fracture often seen with right hand grasp of cyclic (*arrows*)

Postmortem plain film analysis has been helping forensic pathologists for years, [25] however, CT has added much more to the science recently by increasing spatial resolution and detection of projectiles better than ever before [26].

Similar to how trajectories can aid in incident investigation, RAA can add value to aircraft mishap investigation by analyzing injury patterns [27–30]. Folio et al. analyzed a helicopter crash based on the patterns of injury of the pilot in control of the aircraft during impact [31]. Knowing who was on the controls can help the accident board in figuring out potentially preventable human factors issues by looking into crew rest cycles, medications taken, events leading up to the crash, for future prevention of mishaps (when able). In the particular helicopter accident they analyze, the authors believed that RAA helped determine the pilot on the controls at the time of impact. See Fig. 6.36 for plain radiograph of the right hand showing fractures of the first and fifth metacarpals that they believe were the result of the cyclic while the pilot flying was holding firmly. See Fig. 6.37 for artist's depiction of how the fifth metacarpal may have occurred, and Fig. 6.38 for how the first metacarpal may have fractured. Figure 6.39 is a photograph in a military helicopter showing a pilot's hand position on the cyclic for correlation. Figure 6.40a is a gross postmortem photograph of right hand showing echymosis over the first MC from that fracture. Figure 6.40b is a gross postmortem over the area of the fifth MC.

Figure 6.41 shows the left hand and wrist fractures that likely occurred due to holding on of the collective. The collective is always controlled with the left hand, (Fig. 6.41d) and one can see how holding this during impact could result in a fracture dislocation of the left wrist.

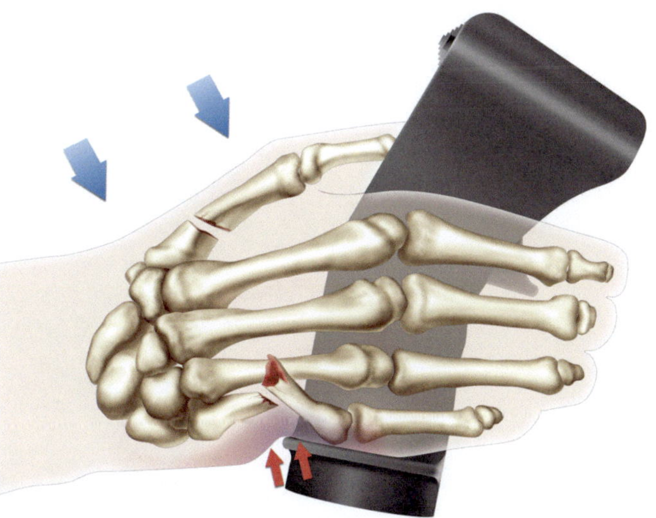

Fig. 6.37 Drawing illustrating how cyclic rest and fifth MC contact during impact

Fig. 6.38 Artist's rendition of thumb and cyclic contact that results in fracture of first MC

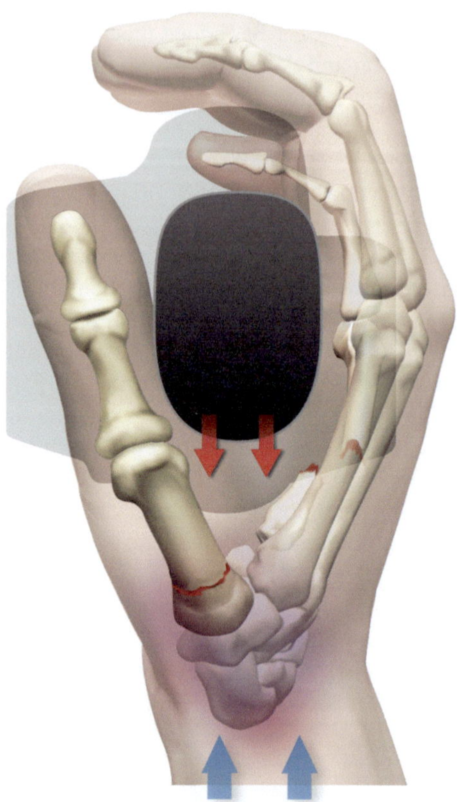

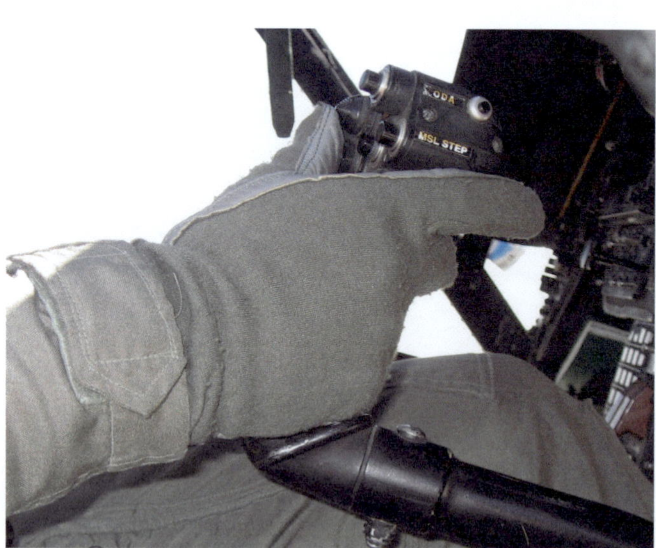

Fig. 6.39 Side photo showing typical hand position relative to cyclic rest. One can see the energy transfer of the fifth MC as it impacts the rest during sudden deceleration and downward force from a crash

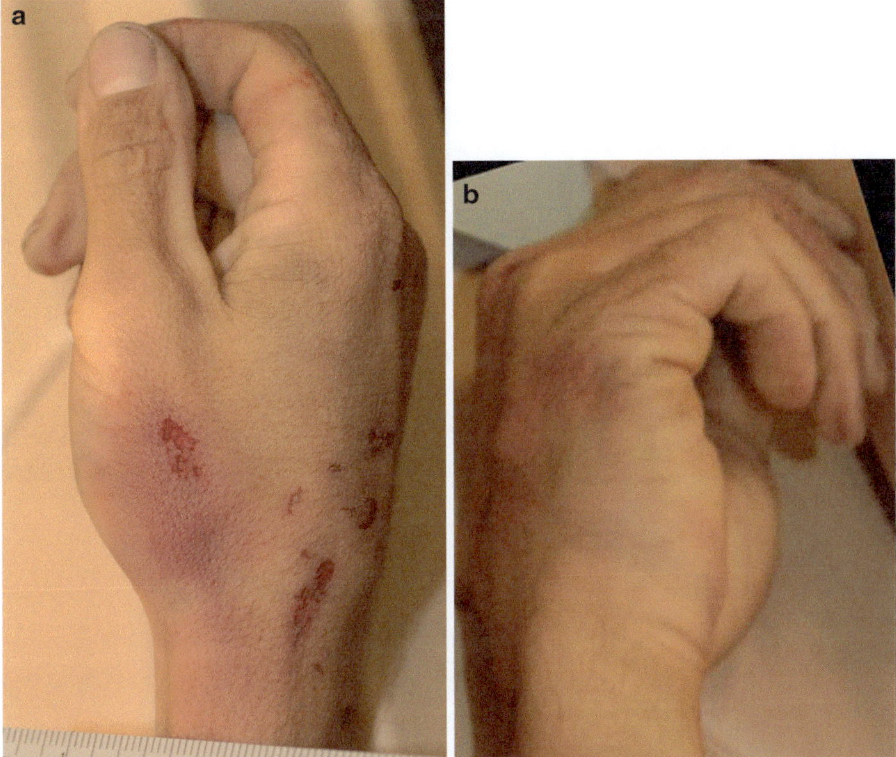

Fig. 6.40 Gross postmortem photograph (**a**) of right hand showing echymosis over the first MC from the fracture likely resulting from the cyclic pressure during impact. Gross autopsy photo (**b**) showing echymosis over fifth MC

This particular mishap demonstrates other clues to direction of impact, occupyable space issues, and cause and manner of death. For example, the Radiology Assisted Autopsy is done with all clothing and gear worn at the time of death; Figs. 6.42 and 6.43 show 3D reconstructions of the head CT with helmet on and digitally subtracted. This way, helmet design and protection efficacy can be evaluated over time, and support for cause of death can be determined by survivability of injury covered in previous chapter. Additionally, a fracture-dislocation of the right hips of both pilots were noted due to cockpit panel contact, not dissimilar to dashboard injuries seen in automobiles. See Figs. 6.44 and 6.45 for pelvis X-ray, 3D CT of pelvis, and artist drawing of injury mechanism and dynamics.

Drawings are by Sofia Echelmeyer and photos are by Dr. Les Folio.

AP Pelvis (Fig. 6.44) and 3D volume rendered reformations (Fig. 6.45) of the pilot presumed at the controls, showing right hip dislocation from secondary impact of cockpit dash. Figure 6.46 shows the dynamics of impact with cockpit panel effects. Note crushing and shearing from sudden deceleration in downward and rightward energy transfer.

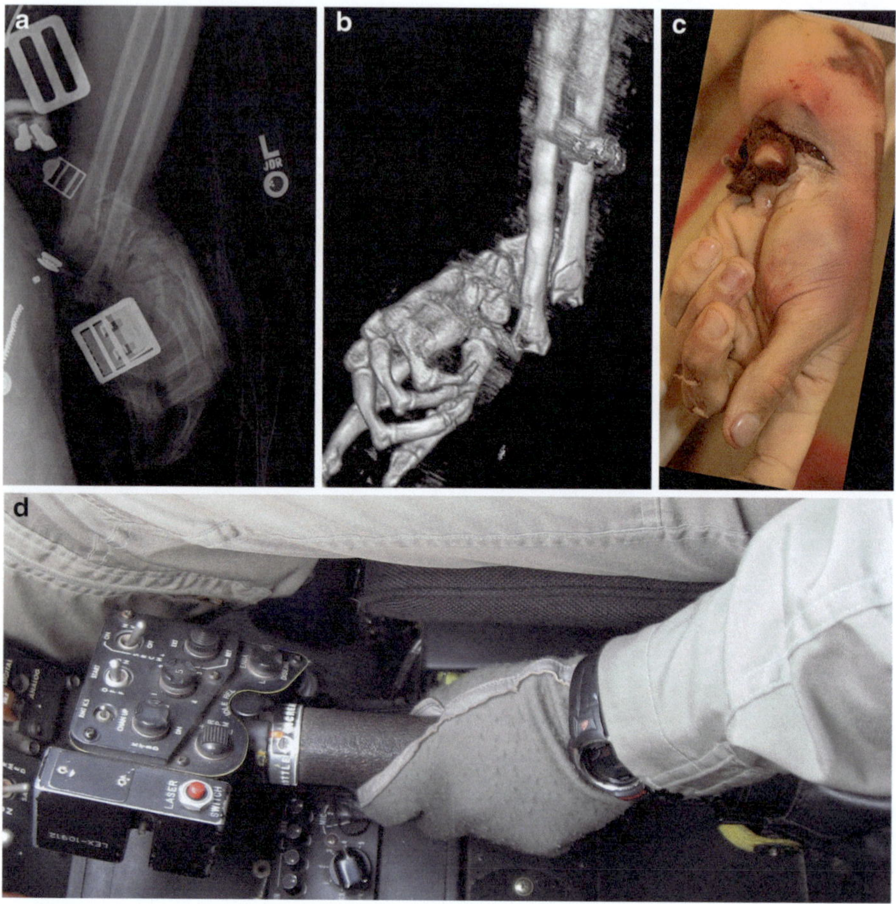

Fig. 6.41 Fracture patterns of left hand and wrist consistent with collective control injury: (**a**) Plain radiography of left hand demonstrating severely displaced open fracture-dislocation of distal radius and ulna. The 3D reformat in (**b**) better illustrates intact distal ulna, with complete dislocation from carpals, and comminuted distal radius fragments severely displaced posteriorly. Gross photo (**c**) from autopsy showing dislocated ulna protruding from open wound. Cockpit photo (**d**) shows typical left hand position on collective

At times in aircraft accidents, there may not be a discernable body or parts left over for investigation. This unfortunate aircraft incident resulted in a few body parts only detected by CT. Following an F-16 crash just off base, a body bag was brought to our hospital for evaluation and was mostly containing aircraft parts that remained from this horrific mishap. See Figs. 6.36 and 6.37 for the AP and lateral CT scouts for the overview of remains. After careful review of the entire axial scans, reformats were attempted to find discernable anatomy for further investigation such as DNA. Figure 6.38 demonstrated what looked to be a phalanx, and was correlated with review at the temporary mortuary in Iraq (Figs. 6.39, 6.47–6.50).

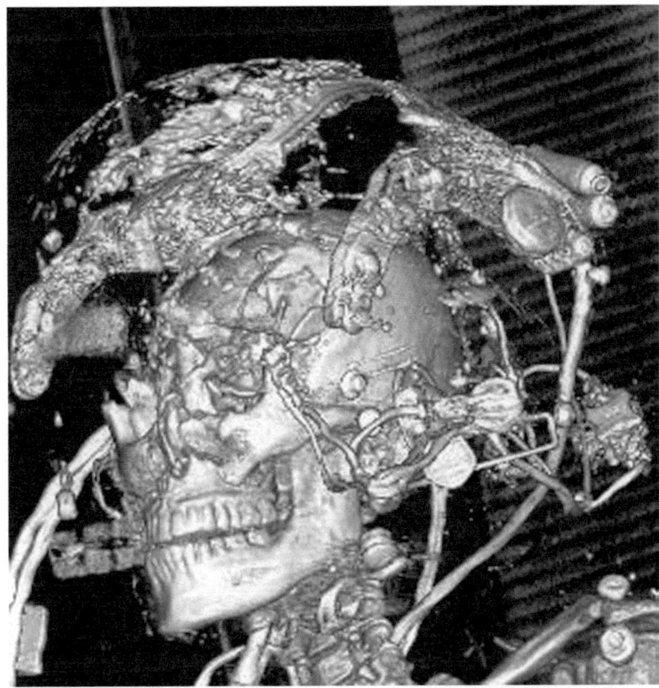

Fig. 6.42 Reformatted images showing the severe skull and facial injuries supporting forward and rightward deceleration blunt injury patterns. Protective gear is imaged in place in hopes to evaluate helmet damage patterns and any associations with cranial patterns

6.8 Summary

Imaging plays an important role in life, limb, and eyesight salvage on the battlefield. Standard reporting formats ensure evaluation of all significant penetrating head injury findings on CT and display pertinent negative findings at a glance. Fast and efficient communication is essential to patient care in the chaotic setting of deployed medicine. More objective severity determination and prognostic indicators on CT may be possible in the near future. This reporting format may be generalizable to busy civilian trauma centers as well. Epidemiologic trends and preventive measures can be better evaluated and refined.

Imaging in eyesight and globe salvageability will likely mature in the near future. Review of existing and future cases of penetrating eye trauma should help narrow the spectrum of salvage determination. Standard report mechanisms can make prospective research on CT grading scales possible for more consistent data mining of standard lexicon.

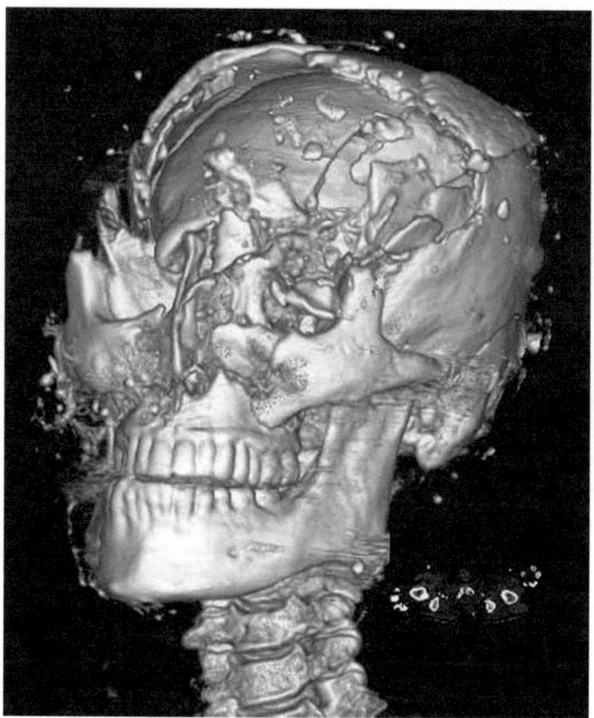

Fig. 6.43 Reformatted images showing the severe skull and facial injuries (with helmet digitally subtracted) supporting forward and rightward deceleration blunt injury patterns. Note the massive disruption of the right zygoma, orbit and frontal bones

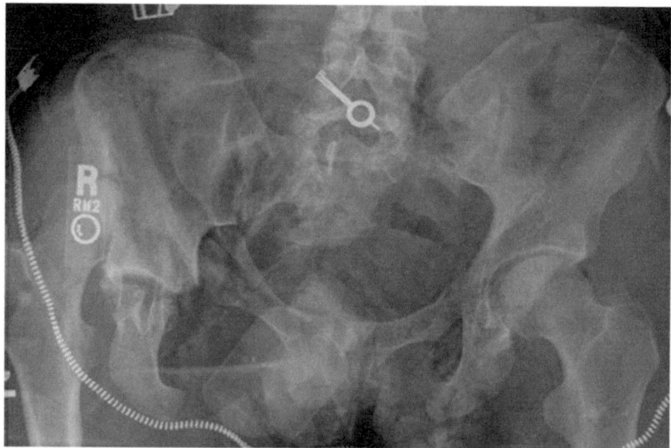

Fig. 6.44 AP pelvis of the pilot presumed at the controls, showing right hip dislocation from secondary impact of cockpit dash

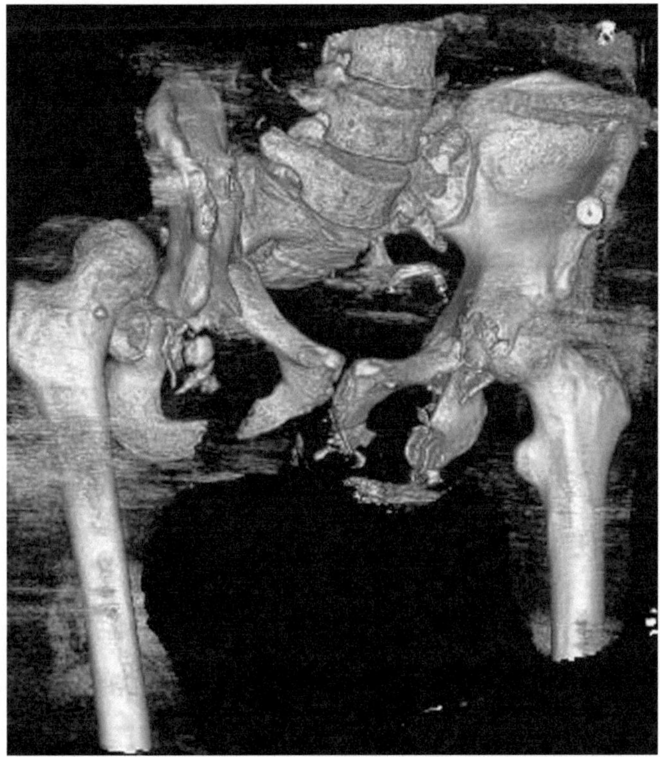

Fig. 6.45 3D volume rendered reformations of the pilot presumed at the controls, showing right hip dislocation from secondary impact of cockpit dash

Blast and ballistic extremity injuries can be evaluated by plain radiography CT and CTA, with determination of severity. CTA of major vessels leading to extremities can be especially helpful in guiding trauma surgeons in triaging these injuries and repairing expeditiously.

Lastly, Radiology Assisted Autopsy (Virtual Autopsy) can be a force multiplier in forensic analysis to help determine cause of death, or cause of life and help medical interventions save more lives in the future; or more importantly, determine the cause of life and help medical interventions save more lives in the future. The unfortunate fatally injured are the heros of medical developments in that the analysis of their injuries will at times help save the lives of those to follow. See Fig. 6.51 for the National Museum of Health and Medicine display on forensic analysis that is doctrine in military medicine. This exhibit is entitled "RESOLVED: Advances in Forensic Identification of US War Dead." This exhibit demonstrates the importance of forensic medicine and the commitment to the identification and commemoration of fatally wounded warriors.

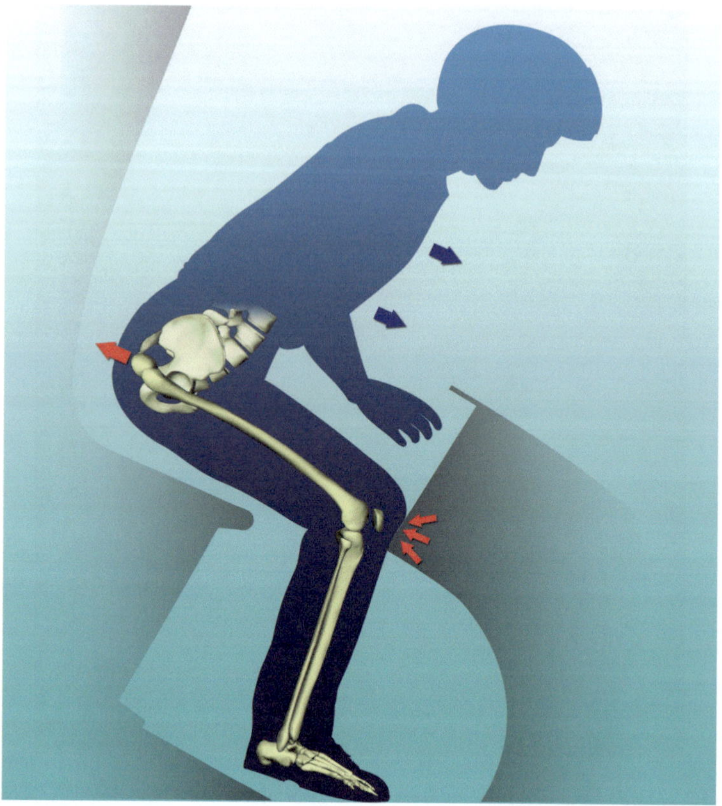

Fig. 6.46 Shows the dynamics of impact with cockpit panel effects. Note crushing and shearing from sudden deceleration in downward and rightward energy transfer

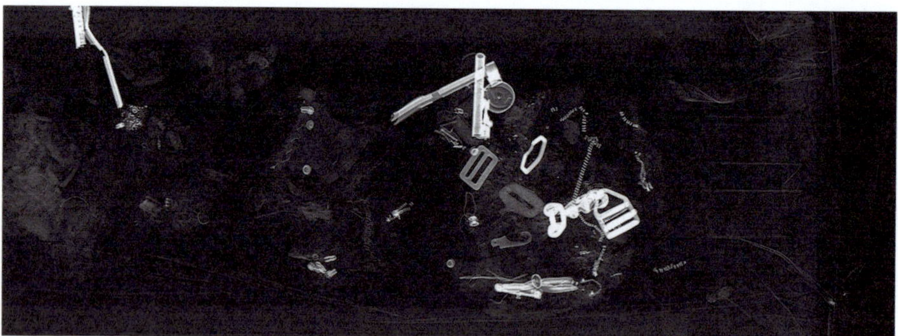

Fig. 6.47 AP CT scout of the only remains salvageable at the site of an F-16 crash where the pilot had no time to eject. No discernable anatomical features were visible on close inspection or plain X-ray

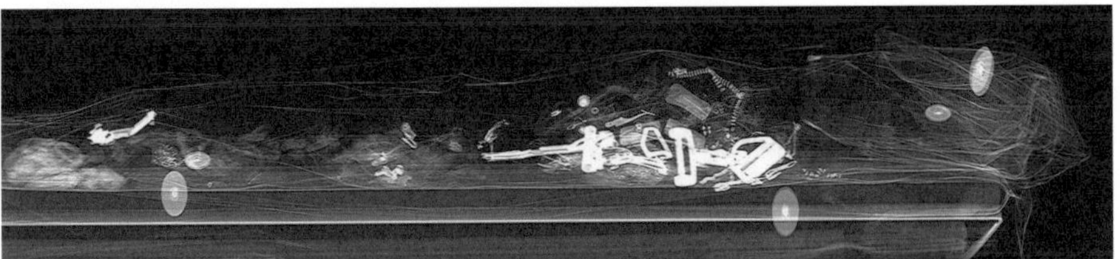

Fig. 6.48 Lateral CT scout again demonstrates mostly aircraft parts rather than recognizable anatomy

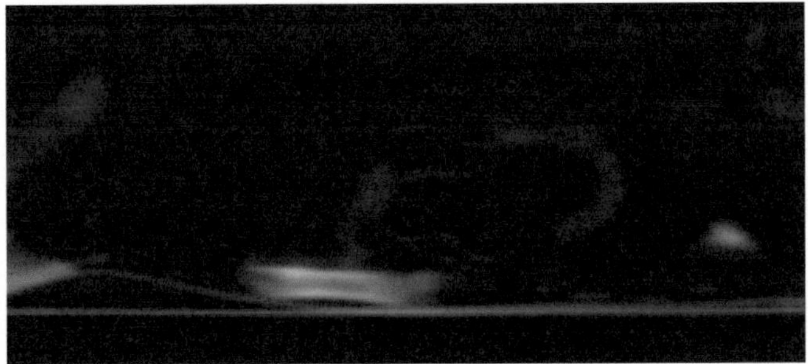

Fig. 6.49 Only after careful review of thin axial slices and reformations was a body part recognized. This lead to closer inspection of the remains in our local mortuary

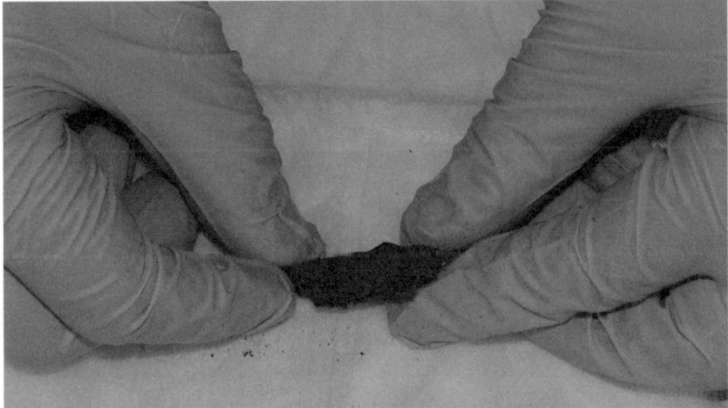

Fig. 6.50 After careful review of the CT, a small phalanx was discovered among the aircraft debris. This was separated for further review back in the US

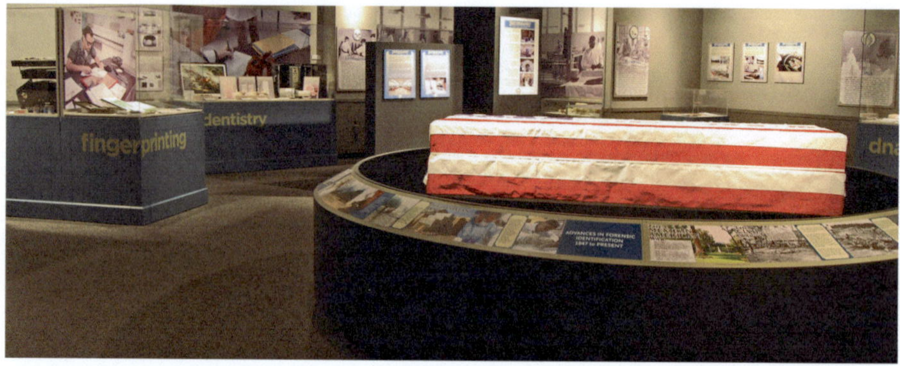

Fig. 6.51 The "RESOLVED: Advances in Forensic Identification of US War Dead" demonstrates the importance of forensic medicine and highlights milestones in forensic identification; from the development of dog tags to DNA analysis and Radiology Assisted Autopsy. In addition to the traditional tools used for positive forensic identification: material evidence, fingerprinting, forensic dentistry, forensic anthropology and forensic pathology, and DNA analysis; Radiology Assisted Autopsy is now routine and mandated in identification of service member and helping determine cause of death (or more importantly, cause of life in future wounded warriors). Donated graciously with permission to reprint by the National Museum of Health and Medicine, Armed Forces Institute of Pathology

Acknowledgments I thank Sofia Echelmeyer for her excellent artwork. I would also like to thank Adrianne Noe, Director at National Museum of Health and Medicine/AFIP, and Tim Clarke, Jr. (Contractor, American Registry of Pathology), Deputy Director (Communications), National Museum of Health and Medicine for donation of the images in this chapter and the first chapter.

References

1. Gowda NK, Agrawal D, Bal C et al. Technetium Tc-99m cysteinate dimer brain single-photon emission ct in mild traumatic brain injury: a prospective study. AJNR Am J Neuroradiol. 2006 Feb; 27:447–451.
2. Ingebrigsten T. Aspects of the management of minor head injury. Tromse University Tromso: Tromprodukt, 1998.
3. Shoung HM, Sichez JP, Pertuiset B. The early prognosis of craniocerebral gunshot wounds in civilian practice as an aid to the choice of treatment. A series of 56 cases studied by the computerized tomography. Acta Neurochir (Wien). 1985; 74(1–2):27–30.
4. Kaufman HH, Loyola WP, Makela ME, Frankowski RF, Wagner KA, Bernstein DP, Gildenberg PL. Civilian gunshot wounds: the limits of salvageability. Acta Neurochir (Wien). 1983; 67(1–2):115–125.
5. Folio LR, Craig S, Singleton B. Emergency decompressive crainiotomy with banked skull flap in subcutaneous pocket. Mil Med. 2006 May/June; 171(5–6):v–viii.
6. Marshall LF, Eisenberg HM, Jane JA et al. A new classification of head injury based on computerized tomography. J Neurosurg. 1991; 75:s14–s20.

7. Marshall LF, Marshall SB, Klauber MR et al. The diagnosis of head injury requires a classification based on computed axial tomography. J Neurotrauma. 1992; 9(Suppl 1):287–292.

8. Guidelines for the management of severe head injury. Brain Trauma Foundation, American Association of Neurological Surgeons, Joint Section on Neurotrauma and Critical Care. J Neurotrauma. 1996; 13:641–734.

9. Vos PE, van Voskuilen AC, Beems T, Krabbe PF, Vogels OJ. Evaluation of the traumatic coma data bank computed tomography classification for severe head injury. J Neurotrauma. 2001 Jul; 18(7):649–655.

10. Meagher S, Galifianakis A, Jannotta D, Krapiva P, Les Folio L. Diffuse axonal injury with negative CT and positive MRI findings. Mil Med. 2008 Nov; 173(11):xx–xxi.

11. Kim KA, Wang MY, McNatt SA, Pinsky G, Liu CY, Giannotta SL, Apuzzo ML.Vector analysis correlating bullet trajectory to outcome after civilian through-and-through gunshot wound to the head: using imaging cues to predict fatal outcome. Neurosurgery. 2005 Oct; 57 (4):737–747.

12. Mackett K, Folio L. CT severity spectrum of penetrating head trauma. American Society of Emergency Radiologists annual meeting. Orlando, FL; October 2009.

13. Abrams E, Folio L. Penetrating eye injuries. Mil Med. 2011 Mar; 176(03).

14. Lemley CA, Wirostko WJ, Mieler WF, McCabe CM, Dieckert JP. Ch 377 Intraocular foreign bodies. In: Albert DM (ed). Principles and Practice of Ophthalmology, 3rd edn. Saunders: Philadelphia, 2008:p 5143.

15. Lemley CA, Wirostko WJ, Mieler WF, McCabe CM, Dieckert JP. Ch 377 Intraocular foreign bodies. In: Albert DM (ed). Principles and Practice of Ophthalmology. 3rd edn. Philadelphia, PA: Saunders, 2008:p 5143.

16. Ehlers JP, Kunimoto DY, Ittoop S, Maguire JI, Ho AC, Regillo CD. Metallic intraocular foreign bodies: characteristics, interventions, and prognostic factors for visual outcome and globe survival. Am J. Ophthalmol. 2008; 146(3):427–433.

17. Spoor TC. Penetrating orbital injuries. In: An Atlas of Ophthalmic Trauma. Mosby: London, 1997:p 117.

18. Chu A, Levine MR. Gunshot wounds of the eye and orbit. Ophthalmic Surg. 1989; 20 (10):729–735.

19. Lemley CA, Wirostko WJ, Mieler WF, McCabe CM, Dieckert JP. Ch 377 Intraocular foreign bodies. In: Albert DM (ed). Principles and Practice of Ophthalmology. 3rd edn. Philadelphia, PA: Saunders; 2008:p 5143.

20. Thach AB, Ward TP, Dick JS II et al. Intraocular foreign body injuries during Operation Iraqi Freedom. Ophthalmology. 2005; 112(10):1829–1833.

21. Colyer MH, Weber ED, Weichel ED et al. Delayed intraocular foreign body removal without endophthalmitis during Operations Iraqi Freedom and Enduring Freedom. Opthalmology. 2007; 114:1439–1447.

22. Ehlers JP, Kunimoto DY, Ittoop S, Maguire JI, Ho AC, Regillo CD. Metallic intraocular foreign bodies: characteristics, interventions, and prognostic factors for visual outcome and globe survival. Am J. Ophthalmol. 2008; 146(3):427–433.

23. Ehlers JP, Kunimoto DY, Ittoop S, Maguire JI, Ho AC, Regillo CD. Metallic intraocular foreign bodies: characteristics, interventions, and prognostic factors for visual outcome and globe survival. Am J Ophthalmol. 2008; 146(3):427–433.

24. Savar A, Andreoli MT, Kloek CE, Andreoli CM. Enucleation for open globe injury. Am J Ophthalmol. 2009; 147(4):595–600.

25. Lichtenstein JE, Fitzpatrick JJ, Madewell JE. The role of radiology in fatality investigations. AJR Am J Roentgenol. 1988 Apr; 150(4):751–755.

26. Harcke HT, Levy AD, Abbott RM, Mallak CT, Getz JM, Champion HR, Pearse L. Autopsy radiography: digital radiographs (DR) vs multidetector computed tomography (MDCT) in high-velocity gunshot-wound victims. Am J Forensic Med Pathol. 2007 Mar; 28(1):13–19.

27. Krefft S. Estimation of pilot control at the time of the crash. In: Mason JK, Reals WJ (eds). Aerospace Pathology. College of American Pathologists Foundation: Chicago, 1973.
28. Krefft S. Who was at the aircraft's controls when the fatal accident occurred? Aerospace Med. 1970; 41(7):785–789.
29. Coltart WD. Aviator's astragalus. J Bone Joint Surg Br. 1952; 34-B(4):545–566.
30. Anderson HG. The Medical and Surgical Aspects on Aviation. Henry Frowde Oxford University Press: London, 1919.
31. Folio L, Harcke T, Luzi S. Radiology-assisted autopsy in helicopter mishap. Aviat Space Environ Med. 2009 Apr; 80(4):400–404.

Chapter 7
Imaging Traumatic Brain Injury
On and Off the Battlefield

Keywords Traumatic brain injury · Diffuse axonal injury · Diffusion tensor imaging · Imaging severity spectrum · Military acute concussion evaluation · Repeatable battery for the assessment of neuropsychological status · Cognitive stability index · Automated neuropsychological assessment metrics · Rubber bullet

7.1 Introduction

Deployed military personnel routinely work in hostile environments with significant exposure to potentially injurious blasts. Traumatic Brain Injury (TBI) secondary to blast has been labeled a signature injury mechanism. Blast injuries are a medical challenge for physicians in recent conflicts, with multiple blast injuries everyday among US military personnel [1]. In the previous chapter, I showed an imaging spectrum of severity in penetrating head injuries as a guide for providers to tailor imaging with clinical suspicion. The majority of Traumatic Brain Injury seen clinically in combat is mild TBI (mTBI). The remaining severity injuries are moderate, severe, and penetrating (that can be further classified mild, moderate, severe) TBI. Mild TBI is injury with loss of consciousness, or altered mental status such as dazed or confused [2], or sometimes referred to as concussion [3].

Until recently, mTBI was not considered to be a structural injury discoverable on CT or MRI. Although mTBI is not consistently detectable on MR or CT, evolving technologies that will be introduced at the end of this chapter are fortunately discovering what was previously not detectable [4].

The mechanism of blasts injuries can be divided into blast displacement and blast overpressure as mentioned in earlier chapters. Judicious use of body armor, reinforced vehicles, and other protective equipment have resulted in a higher survival rate in injured soldiers that would have died of wounds in previous wars from blast injuries [5]. Although these precautions are providing significant life-saving protection against flying fragments and blast displacement, subtle injuries are resulting in relatively higher frequency and often occult to physicians. This is

L. Folio (ed.), *Combat Radiology: Diagnostic Imaging of Blast and Ballistic Injuries*,
DOI 10.1007/978-1-4419-5854-9_7, © Springer Science+Business Media, LLC 2010</p>

important with mTBI that is serious enough to cause neurocognitive changes, however, not currently detectable on traditional CT imaging in theater.

This chapter will focus on closed traumatic head injury, with cases highlighting another spectrum starting with the mildest injury types seen on imaging to the more severe, following a discussion on the clinical and public health perspectives/ challenges of mTBI in combat.

7.2 Clinical and Public Health Considerations in mTBI in Combat

Soldiers, sailors, and airmen exposed to blasts often do not accurately recall how close they were to an explosion, or the importance of effects when no visible physical injuries occur. Like in many sports where head injury is common, it is difficult to determine how severe a head injury needs to be before seeking medical attention. Similar challenges face the ED physician in combat and in any civilian setting.

he ED physician must note any alteration or loss of consciousness as well as posttraumatic amnesia in suspected mTBI [6]. A study by Ryan et al. in 2003 identified physical and cognitive symptoms that were self-reported a few days or weeks after injury in high rates among concussion patients, headaches, dizziness, fatigue, noise and light sensitivity, memory deficits, attention and con-centration deficits, and executive function deficits. Notably, headache and dizzi-ness were reported immediately after injury as well as later in time [7]. In addition, limitations of CT should be known in that CT alone does not rule out mTBI. Some cognitive assessment tests have been used in combat operations, to include the following: Military Acute Concussion Evaluation (MACE), Repeatable Battery for the Assessment of Neuropsychological Status (RBANS), Cognitive Stability Index (CSI), and Automated Neuropsychological Assessment Metrics (ANAM4). Some of these (or other updated versions) are used along with the patient's history, medical symptoms, and physical exam to help evaluate mTBI and guide treatment options.

A physical sign of blast exposure is tympanic membrane rupture from blast overpressure. This injury can occur at low pressures: rupture or perforation can be caused by a pressure as low as 2.5 kg/cm^2 or 245.2 kPa. This value may seem low for an explosive blast, however, from the decibel level perspective it is relatively loud, significantly more than close range rifle and small arms firing [8]. The ear is most vulnerable to overpressure injury, hence may be the only sign from a blast exposure. Tympanic membranes are routinely checked in blast exposed casualties during the physical examination, and history of TM rupture can aid the radiologist when evaluating head CT.

It is important that clinicians ordering MRI at all institutions (not just military) mention mechanism of head injury and other important traumatic history (such as blast, roll-over MVA, etc.). This helps radiologists help providers detect abnormalities earlier and at a less severe level. Sequences can be tailored to find earliest signs of trauma by including GRE, DWI, and even DTI, for example.

Xydakis reports that weapons in combat cause injury exhibit three basic mechanisms, or what he coined the "3 B's of injury": ballistics, blasts, and burns. Another study by Xydakis et al. observed that tympanic membrane pathology was frequently overlooked during treatment due to its understated nature [9]. Blast ear injury ranges from sensorineural acoustic trauma to disruption of middle and inner ear structures. They discovered associations between perforation and loss of consciousness among male US soldiers exposed to blasts in combat zones.

Blast injuries are not the only potential cause of mTBI in the active deployed population, for example, motor vehicle accidents, sports injuries, falls, and fights are also causes, however, much less frequent [10, 11].

7.3 Imaging in TBI

As will be shown here, MRI is more sensitive for detecting mTBI, however, CT remains the diagnostic imaging tool of choice in combat for many reasons. For example, the combat environment is not conducive to MRI and would stress the scanners. In addition, necessary maintenance would not be consistently available. Casualties with metallic gear, unexploded ordinance, and amounts of retained metal fragments would compromise the magnetic field and possibly damage to the patient and scanner.

Basically, other diagnostic tools mentioned here need to be explored until MRI is ready for combat hospitals. Perhaps CT perfusion may help in the future of combat imaging since MR cannot yet be used.

When a provider suspects, mTBI casualties are evacuated to higher echelons of care for MRI with special trauma sequences. Several combat cases previously published are shown here with a variety of negative and positive findings demonstrating a spectrum of severity from most subtle to more severe. The next three cases are well described by Meager et al. for more discussion [12].

As mentioned previously, many patients may express neurological symptoms without CT or MRI findings. Hence, the next level or first imaging level of mTBI is shown here, with a negative CT and only one positive MRI sequence (see Fig. 7.1). This is a 36-year-old male exposed to a blast during combat. The posttraumatic CT in theater was negative. Following evacuation to a higher eschelon of care, an MRI was performed (Fig. 7.2). This gradient echo (GRE) image shows punctate foci of white matter, low signal in the right frontal lobe, and superior aspect of right parietal lobe. The T1 and T2 weighted images did were unremarkable. Meager et al. described these areas of parenchymal hemosiderin deposition likely due to traumatic shearing injury.

The next case is slightly more severe, a 40-year-old man status postblast injury. The CT was again negative (Fig. 7.3), however, the MRI (Fig. 7.4) had a few more foci of decreased signal intensity evident in both hemispheres on gradient echo

Fig. 7.1 Nonenhancing CT fails to demonstrate abnormality. (Reprinted with permission from Military Medicine: International Journal of AMSUS)

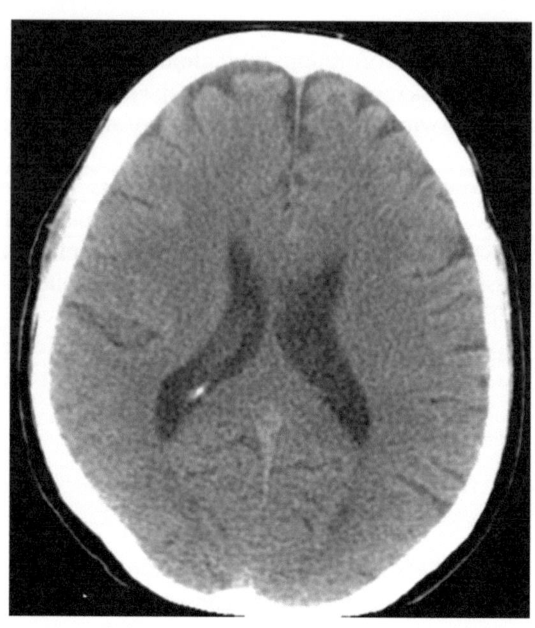

Fig. 7.2 MR Gradient Echo Image in the same patient at the same level demonstrates a focus of low signal in the anterior radiations of the right frontal lobe (*arrow*). This focus represents hemosiderin deposition consistent with shearing injury or diffuse axonal injury. (Reprinted with permission from Military Medicine: International Journal of AMSUS)

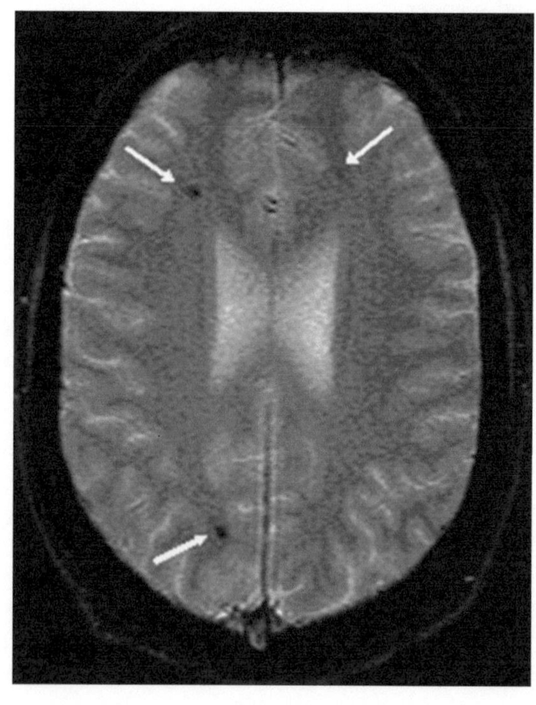

Fig. 7.3 Non-enhancing CT fails to demonstrate abnormality. (Reprinted with permission from Military Medicine: International Journal of AMSUS)

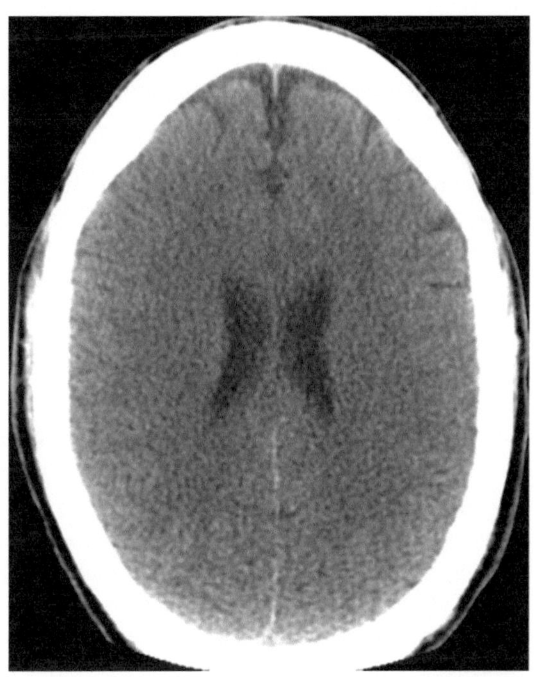

Fig. 7.4 MR Axial GRE (gradient echo, B) image at the corresponding region shows multiple low signal foci, two in the right hemisphere and a less conspicuous focus in the left frontal lobe consistent with hemosiderin deposition (*arrows*). (Reprinted with permission from Military Medicine: International Journal of AMSUS)

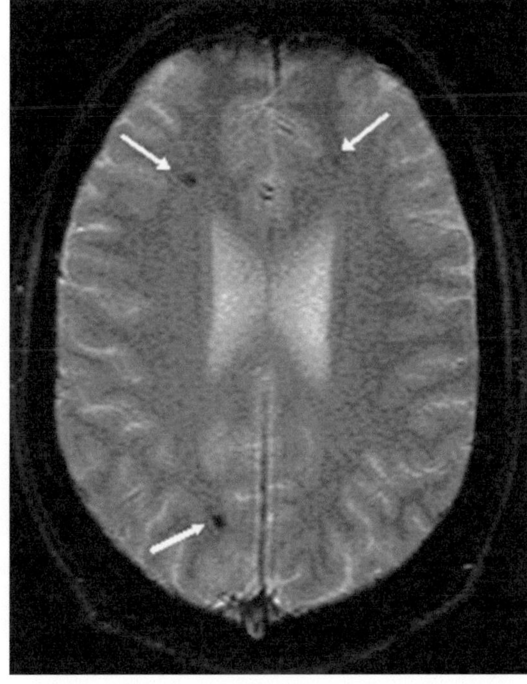

sequences. This again was consistent with hemosiderin deposition at the interface between gray and white matter, DAI.

This last case in Meager's imaging spectrum of mTBI is a 27-year-old male pilot that sustained a closed head injury in a helicopter crash. Noncontrast CT showed intraventricular hemorrhage (Fig. 7.5) and an area of low attenuation in the corpus callosum (Fig. 7.6), and a dense focus in the right frontal lobe (Fig. 7.7). On MRI, these areas were better demonstrated (Figs. 7.8 and 7.9). Other MRI sequences showed findings and available in Military Medicine. These findings are consistent with intraventricular hemorrhage, contusion with a more extensive involvement of Diffuse Axonal Injury than the other two less severe cases.

7.4   Future of Imaging in mTBI due to Blast Injuries

The next case demonstrates the use of DTI (Diffusion Tensor Imaging) in early detection of mTBI. This case is well demonstrated by Rosen et al. [13]. This report is the first where an association was found between conduction aphasia and damage to the AF on the left, and conduction aprosodia and damage to the homologous structure on the right, in a patient who experienced a traumatic brain injury due to a blast. Rosen presents a 23-year-old male that was exposed to two separate blasts in 2004 in close proximity (5 ft).

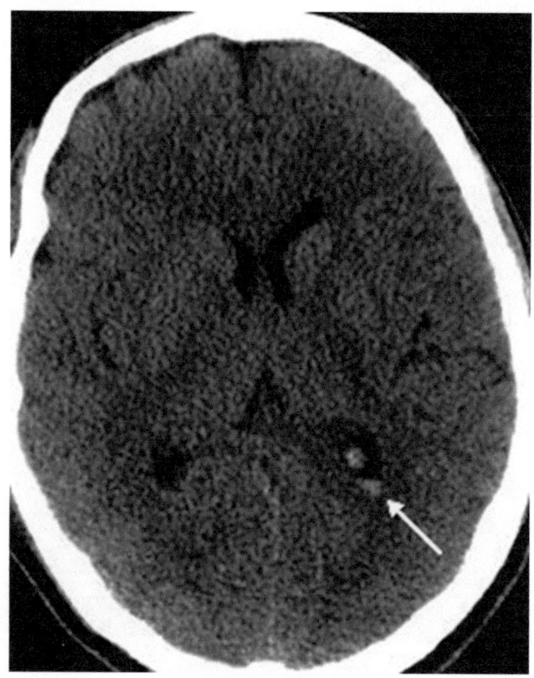

Fig. 7.5 NECT demonstrates dense layering of blood in the posterior horn of the left lateral ventricle (*arrow*)

Fig. 7.6 NECT (A) shows low density area in the callosal parenchyma consistent with edema (*arrow*)

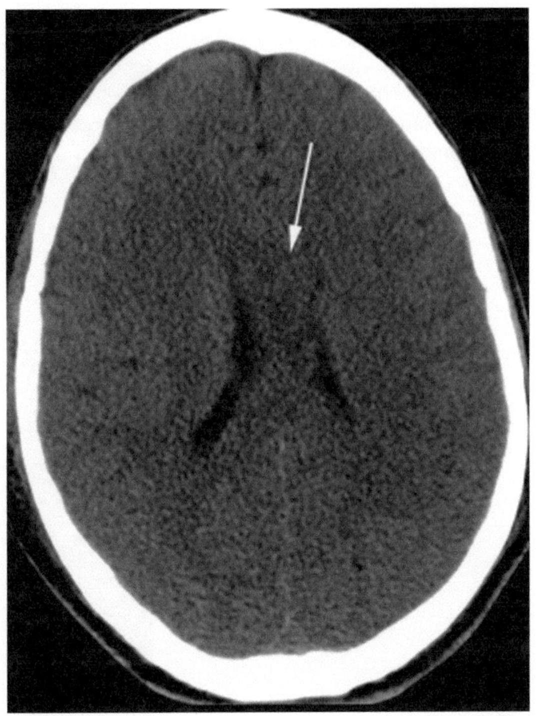

Fig. 7.7 NECT (C) shows small round hemorrhagic focus in the right frontal lobe (*arrow*)

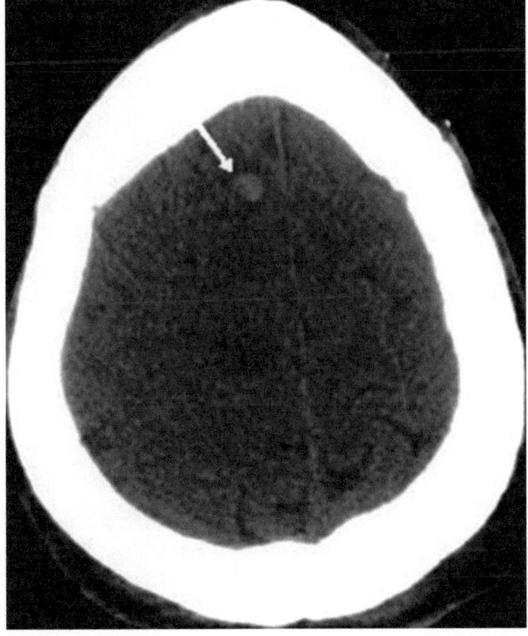

Fig. 7.8 Axial GRE again showing layering blood, now seen (due to increased sensitivity of MR) in both posterior horns (*arrows*), left more than right

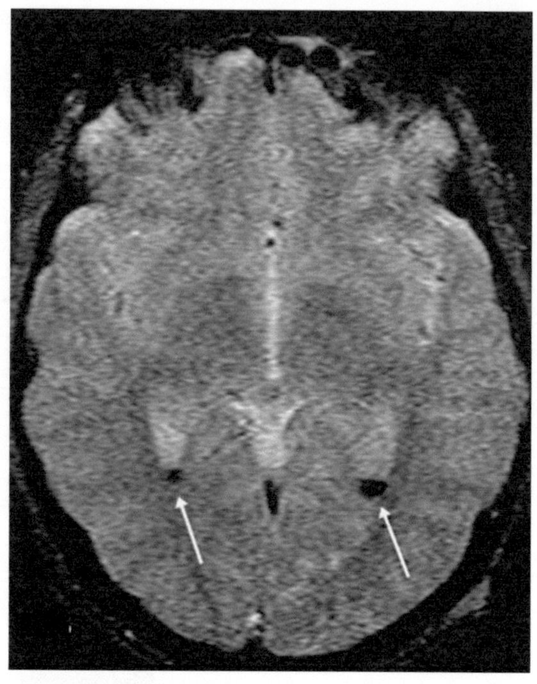

Fig. 7.9 DWI sequence (C) shows restricted diffusion at the same level (*arrow*)

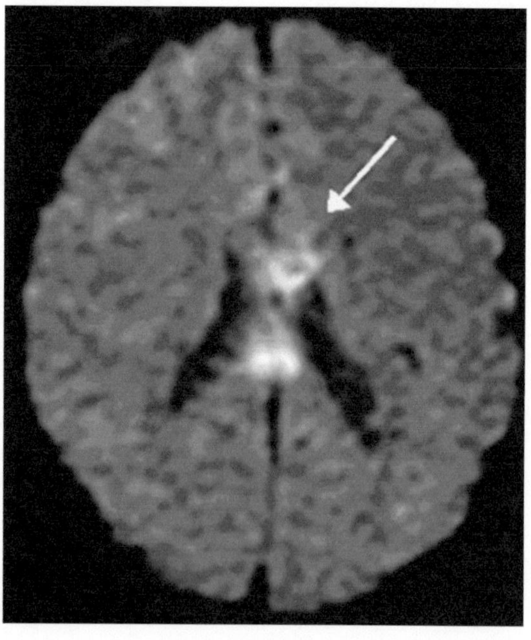

Two months after the first blast, he was exposed to a second blast and then reported headaches, intermittent tinnitus without hearing loss, and a conduction aphasia on the Boston Diagnostic Aphasia examination. The patient had an MRI with DTI and a PET scan. The CT was negative.

The DTI tractography (Fig. 7.10) was positive for fiber thinning of the Arcuate Fasciculus, see Fig. 7.11 for a normal Arcuate Fasciculus.

Conventional MRI (1.5 Tesla, without DTI) was negative. A PET showed subtle asymmetry in the left temporal region. A 4-Tesla MRI with DTI and tractography of the left AF and its homologue on the right (Fig. 7.10) was done soon after the clinical MR (March 2007).

The DTI 4 months later after intensive speech and language therapy and tractography was similar with slight sprouting around the locations that appeared to have

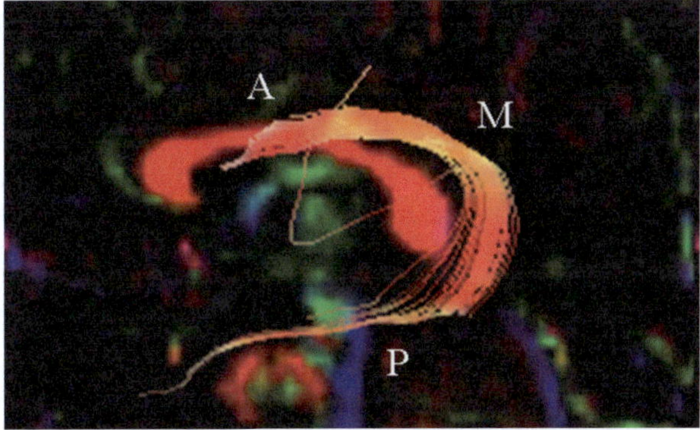

Fig. 7.10 DTI demonstrating left Arcuate Fasciculus (in *orange*) of patient showing that the fiber tract is much thinner than that of the normal (Fig. 7.11 below). A is the anterior portion of the Arcuate Fasciculus (*M* middle; *P* posterior). (Reprinted with permission from Military Medicine: International Journal of AMSUS)

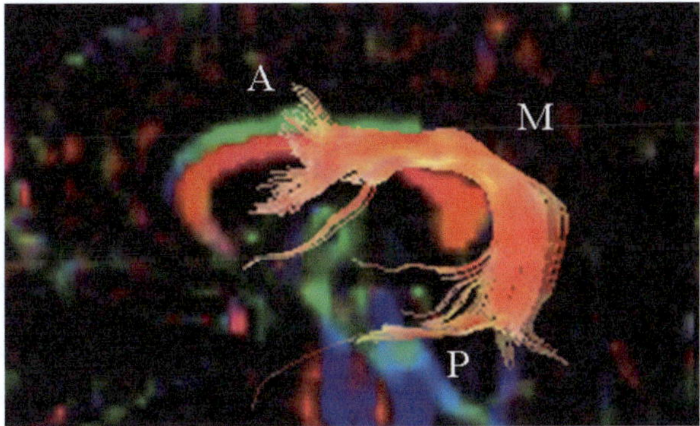

Fig. 7.11 Normal DTI of same region and same perspective for comparison. (Reprinted with permission from Military Medicine: International Journal of AMSUS)

been sheared, particularly on the left side, see Rosen article for images and more discussion. These findings were consistent with Arcuate Fasciculus Damage in a blast-exposed soldier with mild traumatic brain injury (mTBI) and associated conduction aphasia.

7.5 Summary of Closed Head Injury and mTBI Imaging

Evolving imaging advances may redefine imaging findings in mTBI in the near future. The cases presented here show how GRE, DWI, and DTI can increase sensitivity of detection on MR. Application of DTI, 3T MRI, and temporal lobe volume imaging may help increase sensitivity and is worthy of further investigation. A recent study with 3T MRI is promising in detecting mTBI [14]. For example, trauma has been shown to result in white matter loss and hippocampal atrophy. There may be useful imaging corollaries between neurodegenerative changes and mTBI. In addition, trauma changes morphometric temporal lobe relationships and is associated with poorer memory performance [15]. On the other end of the cognitive spectrum, one study demonstrated that taxi drivers in London had greater gray matter volume than controls (bus drivers) in mid-posterior hippocampi and less volume in anterior hippocampi due to more demand on navigational spatial orientation [16, 17]. London taxi drivers have stringent requirements and periodic testing of location knowledge, routes, and even hospital locations and capabilities. This indicates that there is a capacity for local plastic change in the healthy adult brain in response to environmental demands. Sensitivity of volumetric MRI could therefore be promising in detecting early changes in mTBI.

7.6 Penetrating TBI

Delving into the more extreme head injuries, a few more cases are illustrated. Other cases are available in other chapters of this book and some published cases. The following case shows how a riot control weapon can cause damage if directed at the right anatomic region. This individual was being chased by police and would not halt; so they shot him in the face on the right. See Figs. 7.12 and 7.13 for an example of a rubber bullet on CT.

This last case demonstrates a penetrating injury from a large knife in an active-duty deployed soldier. He was in a close-range firefight and stabbed in the side of the head. On arrival to our combat hospital, he was awake and alert and remembered the incident. He was neurologically intact with 5/5 strength in all four extremities and GCS of 15. See Fig. 7.14 for 3D of knife position in head. Figure 7.15 shows the intracranial knife blade in close proximity to petrous ICA. Axial MIP in bone windows (Fig. 7.16) also shows the knife relationship that can

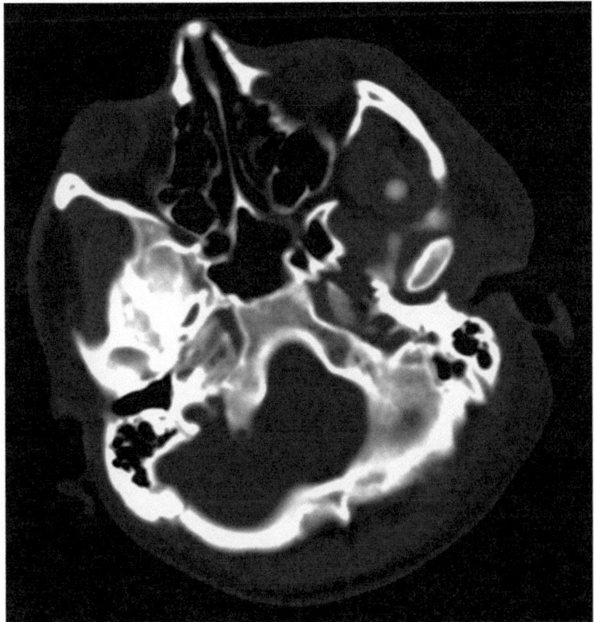

Fig. 7.12 CT bone windows showing rubber bullet just inside of zygomatic arch

help the neurosurgeon navigate. Axial CT (Fig. 7.17) shows a right subdural hematoma with midline shift. Figure 7.18 shows the operative preparation photo with the knife in the side of the head.

7.7 TBI Treatment

There are many recent advances in TBI treatment. Decompressive Craniotomy has been a mainstay of severe penetrating head injury in current conflicts. It allows immediate room for swelling while improving intracerebral blood flow. An interesting surgical craniotomy technique was developed at the onset of the recent campaign in Iraq for more severe injuries to immediately relieve intracranial swelling following a blast while preserving the portion of skull removed [18]. This involves taking the removed skull flap, implanting it into the abdomen temporarily to allow for adequate blood flow, and easy access for recovery and replacement later. This keeps the patient's own bone viable. Stereolithography from CT data is now used to digitally reconstruct the patient's skull and custom design materials that can be used in cranial reconstruction [19].

Once the medical profession becomes more familiar with penetrating head injury to include blast effects and available medical resources (time, blood, staff, surgical capabilities), analysis may be better estimated by determining survivable versus nonsurvivable (expectant) CT findings, as well as predictability for quality

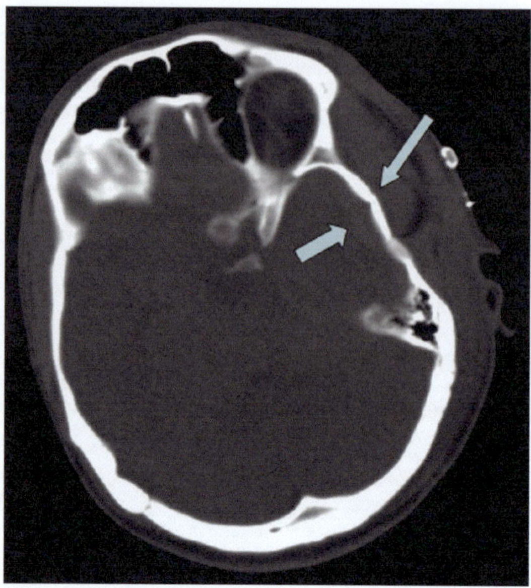

Fig. 7.13 CT more superior showing impact point of rubber bullet causing both a temporal bone fracture and small epi-axial collection of blood. Only superficial exploration was necessary with antibiotics

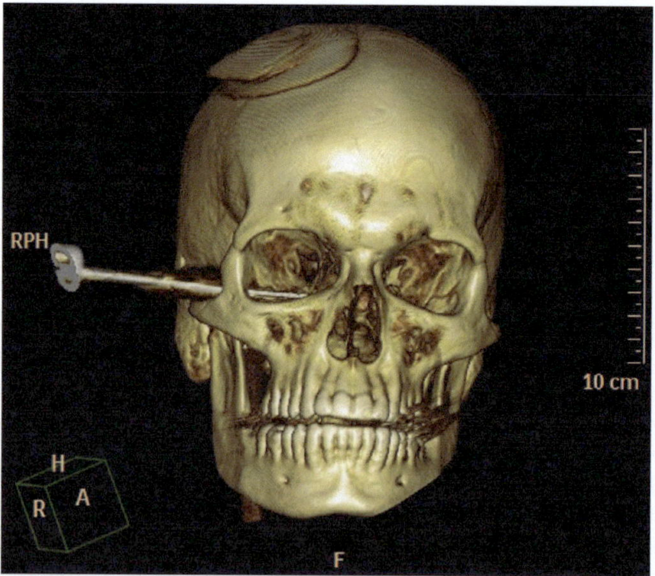

Fig. 7.14 CT 3D demonstrating the relationship of the knife to the zygoma and orbit (reprinted with permission from Military Medicine: International Journal of AMSUS)

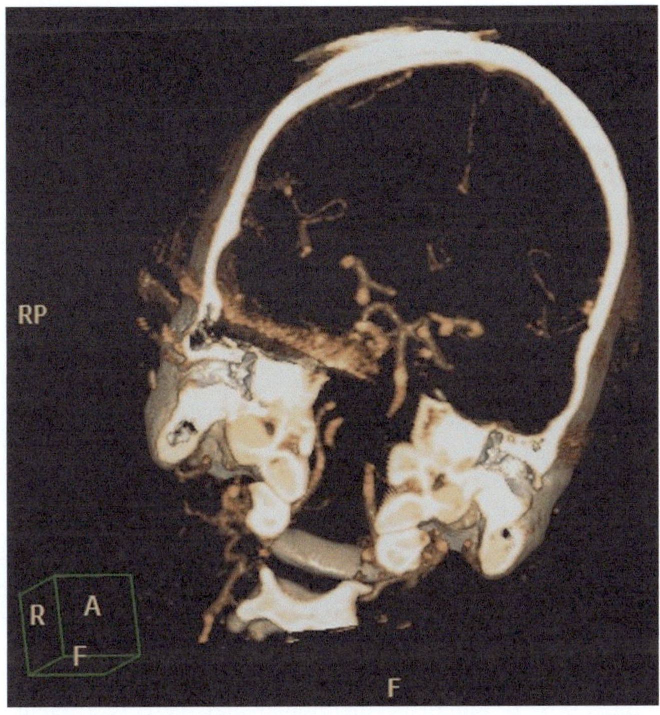

Fig. 7.15 CTA coronal MIP showing the knife relationship to intracranial vessels. The knife traverses the path of the distal R petrous ICA below the take off of the R othalmic artery. There was no extravasation seen. However, transaction was a concern (reprinted with permission from Military Medicine: International Journal of AMSUS)

Fig. 7.16 Axial MIP again demonstrating intracranial portion of knife. (Reprinted with permission from Military Medicine: International Journal of AMSUS)

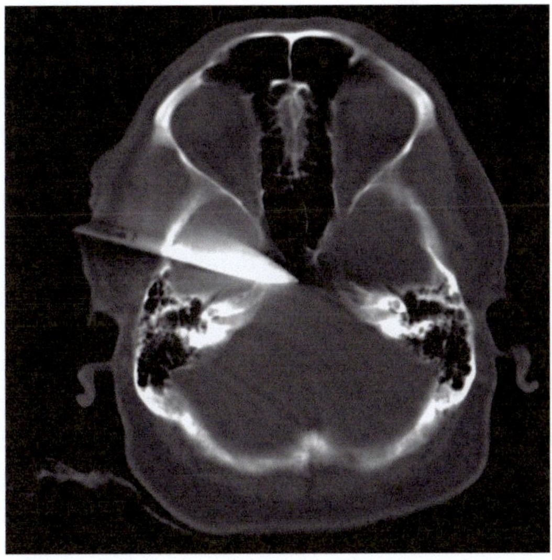

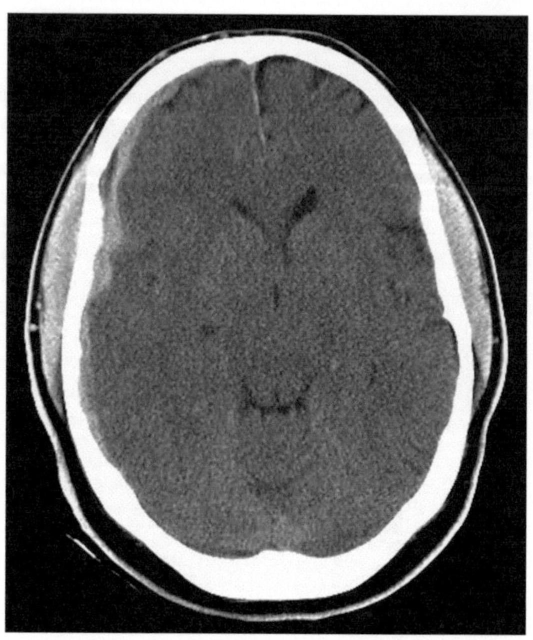

Fig. 7.17 CT axial showing a 1 cm of L midline shift and a 1 cm thick right subdural hematoma (reprinted with permission from Military Medicine: International Journal of AMSUS)

of life determinations. It should be mentioned that there is a telemedicine tool available for military providers for questions about TBI in general. Questions can be emailed to tbi.consult@us.army.mil by any military service. Although this is an Army email, AF, PHS, and Navy (and VA) can email with questions.

7.8 Summary

This chapter demonstrated a closed-head injury imaging spectrum of TBI from mild to severe. Cases of TBI were presented starting with the most subtle findings (negative CT, positive MR on one sequence only) to the more severe (positive CT and MR on multiple sequences). The more severe open penetrating and perforating head injury (such as dural compromise from skull or facial bone fracture) was covered in the previous chapter. Together, this spectrum of cases should help put the imaging severity scale in perspective for future research on extensions of grading and predictability. Survivability surrogates or CT grading of penetrating trauma may be able to be determined after review of consistent data collected from recent deployed experience through accurate, detailed data recording. Although a

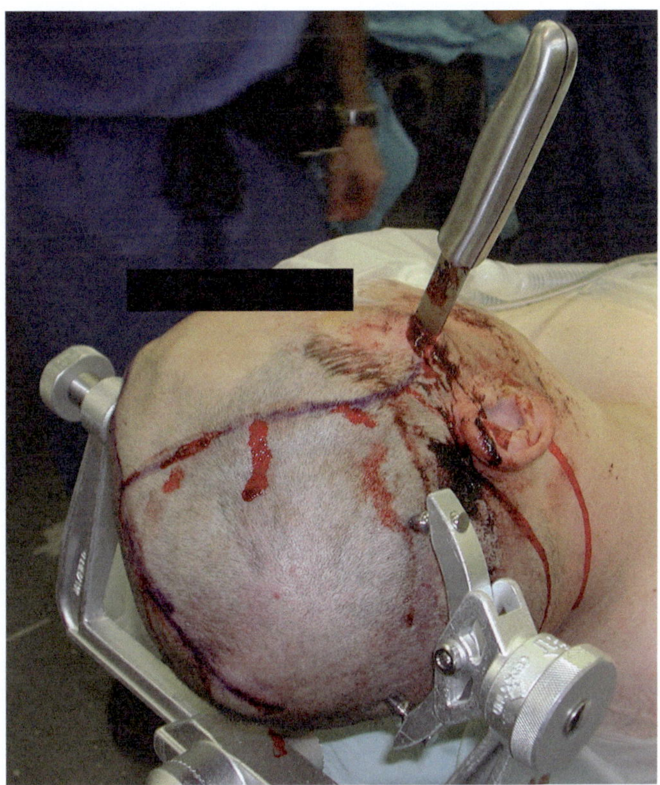

Fig. 7.18 Operative photo demonstrating the knife location. A frontotemporoparietal craniectomy was performed. When the knife was removed, there was a great deal of intradural and extradural bleeding. An intraoperative direct ICA angiogram failed to demonstrate ICA extravasation. (Reprinted with permission from Military Medicine: International Journal of AMSUS)

succinct score such as a "CT GCS" is not likely anytime soon, this is not an impossible future concept to consider based on clinical record review, more standard and objective CT reports (discussed in further detail and organized below), and mechanism of injury.

This should provide a baseline of knowledge of diagnostic imaging utilization in the current conflicts and traumatic brain injury in general with evolving transformational technologies. Knowing more about how different modalities and specific sequences identify certain levels of injury can help providers order imaging more effectively.

Fig. 7.19 KUB
demonstrating the
transplanted (temporary)
skull flap within the abdomen
for patient transport from
overseas

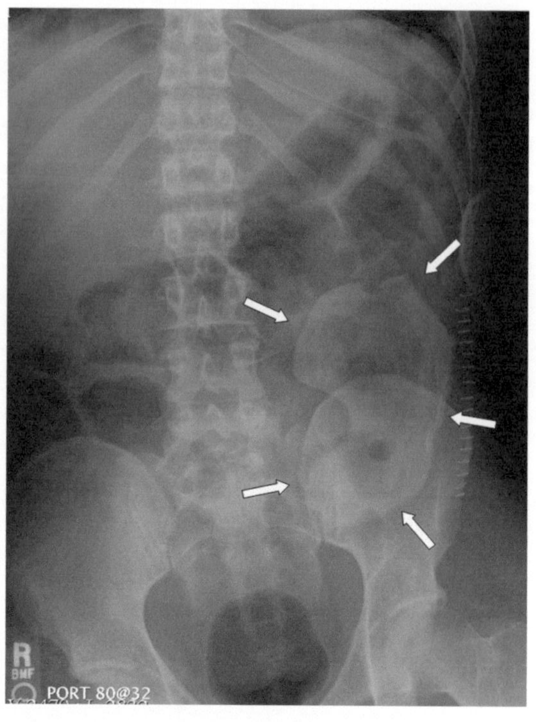

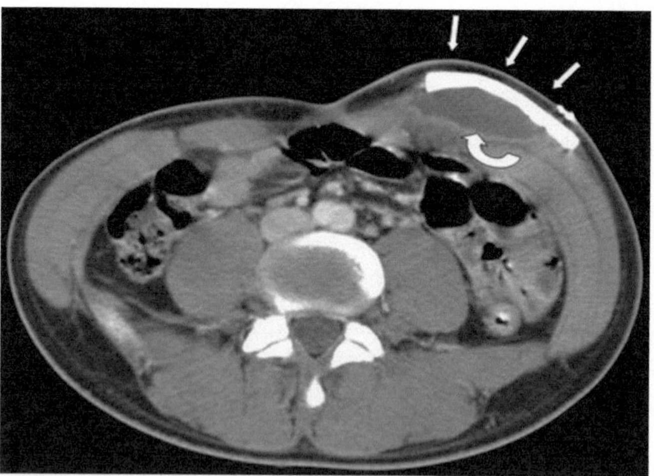

Fig. 7.20 Skull flap seen as bone density in anterior subcutaneous fat (*arrows*). Note fluid
collection representing likely abscess

Fig. 7.21

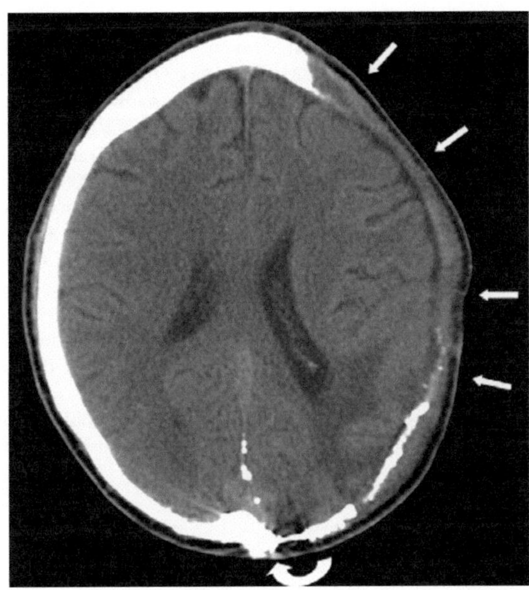

References

1. Xydakis MS et al. Tympanic-membrane perforation as a marker of concussive brain injury in Iraq. N Engl J Med. 2007; 357(8):830–31.
2. Hoge CW et al. Mild traumatic brain injury in U.S. Soldiers returning from Iraq. N Engl J Med. 2008; 358(5):453–63.
3. Defense and veterans brain injury center working group on the acute management of mild traumatic brain injury in military operational settings, clinical practice guideline and recommendations. http://www.dvbic.org (Accessed on 2009 Dec).
4. Hammoud DA, Wasserman BA. Diffuse axonal injuries: pathophysiology and imaging. Neuroimaging Clin N Am. 2002; 12(2):205–16.
5. Okie S. Traumatic brain injury in the war zone. N Engl J Med. 2005; 352(20):2043–47.
6. Sherer M et al. Comparison of indices of TBI severity: Glasgow coma scale, length of coma, post-traumatic amnesia. J Neurol Neurosurg Psychiatry. 2008; 79(6):678–85.
7. Ryan LM, Warden DL. Post concussion syndrome. Int Rev Psychiatry. 2003; 15(4):310–36.
8. Tontechnik-Rechner, Sengpielaudio. Online Sound Unit Conversion Program. http://www.sengpielaudio.com/calculator-soundlevel.htm (Accessed on 2009 Dec).
9. Xydakis MS et al. Analysis of battlefield head and neck injuries in Iraq and Afghanistan. Otolaryngol Head Neck Surg. 2005; 133(4):497–504.
10. Injury update, A report to Oklahoma injury surveillance participants, Nov 7, 1995. http://www.health.state.ok.us/program/Injury/updates/falltbi.html (Accessed on 2009 Dec).
11. Meagher RJ, WF Young. Subdural hematoma, eMedicine, Nov 2, 2006. http://www.emedicine.com/NEURO/topic575.htm (Accessed on 2009 Dec)
12. Meagher S, Galifianakis A, Jannotta D, Krapiva P, Folio L. Diffuse axonal injury with negative CT and positive MRI Findings. Mil Med. 2008 Nov; 173(11):xx–xxi.
13. Rosen A, Zhang Y, Zhan W, Kasprisin A, Martinson S, Cheng J, Weiner M, Yesavage JA, Folio L, Ashford JW. Mild traumatic brain injury and conduction aphasia from a close

   proximity blast resulting in arcuate fasciculus damage diagnosed on DTI tractography. Mil
   Med. 2009 Sept; 174(11):v–vi.
14. Lee H, Wintermark M, Gean AD, Ghajar J, Manley GT, Mukherjee P. Focal lesions in acute
   mild traumatic brain injury and neurocognitive outcome: CT versus 3T MRI. J Neurotrauma,
   2008 Sep; 25(9):1049–56.
15. Bigler ED, Andersob CV, Blatter DD. Temporal lobe morphology in normal aging and
   traumatic brain injury. Am J Neuroradiol. 2002 February; 23:255–66.
16. Maguire EA, Woollett K, Spiers HJ, London taxi drivers and bus drivers: a structural MRI and
   neuropsychological analysis. Hippocampus. 2006; 16(12):1091–101.
17. Maguire EA, Gadian DG, Johnsrude IS, Good CD, Ashburner J, Frackowiak RS, Frith CD.
   Navigation-related structural change in the hippocampi of taxi drivers. Proc Natl Acad Sci U S
   A. 2000; 97(8):4398–403.
18. Folio L, Craig SH, Singleton B. Answer to last month's radiology case and image: emergency
   decompressive craniotomy with banked skull flap in subcutaneous pocket. Mil Med. 2006;
   171(6):vii–viii.
19. Kermer C et al. Preoperative stereolithographic model planning for primary reconstruction in
   craniomaxillofacial trauma surgery. J Craniomaxillofac Surg. 1998; 26(3):136–39.

Chapter 8
Chest Imaging in a Battlefield Hospital

Keywords Blast lung injury · Chest radiology rounds · Hummvee · Barotrauma

8.1   Introduction

The chest X-ray is the bread and butter of diagnostic imaging and among the most common radiologic studies throughout the world, and the combat hospital is no exception. Chest CT is also common in the battlefield hospitals, and not just for initial trauma, but for follow-up trauma (anywhere in the body), the ICU patients, wards, etc., as well. The chest is one of the major indicators of clinical status, and portable CXRs are done almost daily on every ICU patient. Checking the status of tubes and lines, aeration, atelectasis, effusions, contusions, other fluid collections on morning CXR's is a daily activity in combat hospitals, not unlike many civilian hospital ICUs stateside and internationally.

8.2   Chest X-Rays in the Combat Hospital

Like any trauma center or emergency department, the CXR is the first radiological exam (other than FAST) performed. Along with the pelvis and the cervical spine (that is more often covered by a CT), it is the ATLS and hospital doctrine, and for good reasons. In penetrating trauma (not just chest), the CXR can be the imaging indicator for immediate trauma surgery. In hemodynamically unstable patients, it may be the only radiology imaging they get before emergent surgery.

8.3   ICU Chest X-Ray

Chest imaging rounds occurred every morning 7 days a week; without exception in our reading room tent. If rounds were rushed or missed by key staff, it was quickly realized at this daily gathering of the masterminds. The ICU rounds starting with

L. Folio (ed.), *Combat Radiology: Diagnostic Imaging of Blast and Ballistic Injuries,*
DOI 10.1007/978-1-4419-5854-9_8, © Springer Science+Business Media, LLC 2010

morning CXR is many hospitals doctrine. This began the follow-on patient rounds and provided a pulse of the entire hospital. One challenge of the rounds is mornings are busy times with shift changes, meetings, and rounds. As the radiology department chair, I also had to attend morning administrative meetings, some daily, some weekly. Like anywhere else, a leader must sharpen the saw while cutting with it. This took overlap with tired radiologists, and we were lucky enough to have three. Prior rotations were not so lucky and had to endure even more exhausting hours in combat conditions to meet the morning CXR rounds. My conversations and prior visits with radiologists that worked during those times made me feel lucky. Mornings seem to be when everyone wants a piece of you, and like in private practice, there is only so much of you to go around.

We never used Swan–Ganz catheters, we simply did not have the need, nor the time in our population. We used the CXR, CT scout CXR, vitals and basic indicators for life and death, with no chronic care. Hospital stays were hours or days, not weeks, thanks to the excellent Air-Evacuation system mentioned earlier in this book.

Other common conditions seen on CXRs not shown in this book include the usual evaluations of tubes and lines, chest CTA to rule out PE, empyemas, abscesses, lung drainage and catheter follow-up, and E-FAST of the pericardium and pneumothorax.

Several chest trauma cases have been described in prior chapters; I will present additional cases not covered previously and some basic chest plain images that are representative of chest imaging in combat hospitals.

8.4 Imaging Techniques

For penetrating injuries potentially involving the subclavian arteries or other great vessels near the neck and chest, the arm opposite the penetration is injected when possible. This minimizes beam hardening artifact from contrast concentration in the brachiocephalics near the potential damaged vessels. As mentioned earlier in this book, it was not uncommon to use the CT scout to capture traditional plain film studies such as extremities or chest to save time in the imaging process, or to minimize patient movement. If a patient was stable and did not need a chest X-ray to check ET tube position, the CT scout was easily obtained in lieu of the chest X-ray; there was simply no enough time to do otherwise. The quality of the scouts was often acceptable for other anatomic regions, especially if this could save time. Lateral scouts were done routinely, although often limited, they did provide an orthogonal view for spatially localizing metal fragments for example [1]. This maximized imaging resource efficiency in trauma surges and expedited throughput.

8.5 Blast Lung Injury

I would like to start off with the more unique situation of Blast Lung Injury (BLI) since this was unfortunately a daily routine for us during one of the busiest combat operations in Iraq. We have seen other primary blast effects to include hollow organ injury due to overpressure and, secondary blast effects, or the direct effects of debris (see Chap. 3 on types of blasts). Blast lung is the second most common manifestation of primary organ damage in blast injuries. Since BLI is likely often a combination of the types of blast injures (predominately primary and secondary) mentioned in Chap. 3, I will use a separate system for organizing BLI here. Although BLI has been described for years, I believe it has a lot to be yet discovered.

In my experience, there seems to be three patterns of BLI depending on proximity, thoracic mechanical pressure, confined space, airway, and body aspect to the blast origin. We often see BLI as diffuse focal or generalized peripheral or central airspace opacities, distribution often relating the proximity, surroundings, and aspect of the blast.

For organizational purposes, I will divide up the three types of blast lung as airway, generalized overpressure/compression, and focal. A fourth category could be added as a combination of all three; however, many seem to fit this category, but usually have one predominate feature to fit in the other three.

8.5.1 Airway BLI

One cause of BLI is thought to be due to the pressure differential across the alveolar-capillary interface [2] since pulmonary injury can be sustained without evidence of external thoracic injury. Perhaps, the blast overpressure wave can be likened to the extreme pressure differential and explosive potential of extreme pressure differences in a tornado. In some cases, however, a more peripheral and more direct compression effect seems to occur when the pressure wave carries sufficient force to compress the chest wall [3]. Sometimes, this occurs posteriorly against the spine, similar to blunt force injury as seen in MVA and falls. The result in confined space (vehicle or small rooms) or direct airway impact is a transient elevation in intrathoracic pressure – perhaps, a combination of both external thoracic pressure and forced airway pressure for BLI, depending again on proximity, surroundings, type of blast, etc.

One classic imaging finding in pulmonary barotraumas from overpressure forced air is described as a bihilar "butterfly" pattern consistent with pulmonary contusion. Additional findings may include localized pulmonary contusion, pneumothorax, and hemothorax among others [4]. With severe cases, pulmonary lacerations and pneumatoceles can develop, some tearing likely to alveolar over distention [5, 6]. Elastic recoil [7] and shearing effects may be responsible for these resultant alveolar and parenchymal tears.

This first case demonstrates the central airspace distribution of consolidations, to include central parenchymal tears, likely representing a direct airway pressure in light of the injury occurring directly to the mouth and nose. In this case, a Rocket Powered Grenade (RPG) blew up near the casualty's nose and mouth, see Fig. 8.1 for 3D of resulting facial fractures. The lung CT (Figs. 8.2 and 8.3) showed

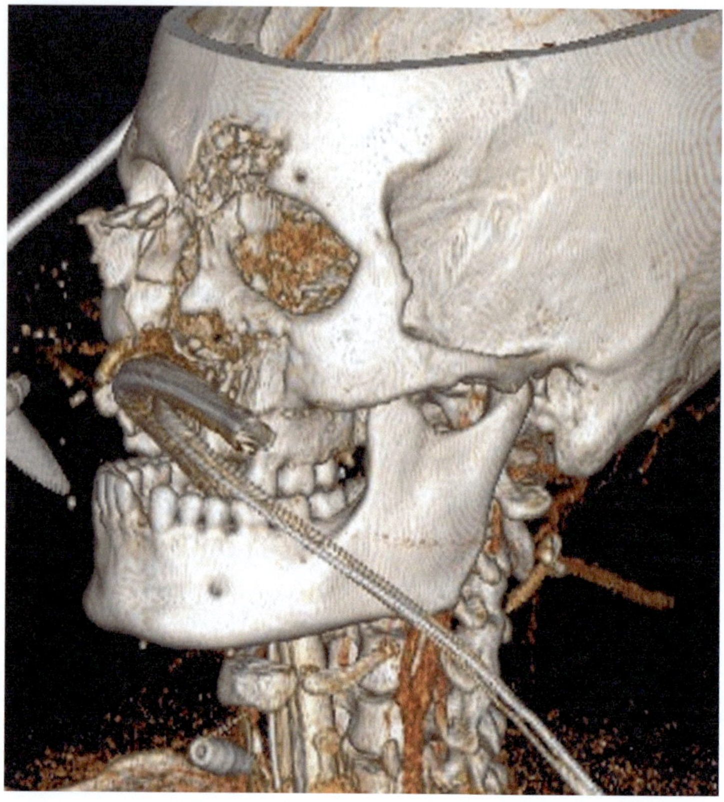

Fig. 8.1 RPG verses none and mouth. The 3D volume rendered images of the face represent central facial fractures (focal facial smash) from explosion in close proximity to the blast

lucencies consistent with central parenchymal tears. This was correlated positively with respiratory monitoring with pressure graphs appearing like emphysematous bleb rupture and flap effect.

Another unusual situation in blast injuries is blast particle aspiration when in close range of an explosion. This next case highlights aspiration of sand directly into the lung seen in upper airways on CT. Direct particle aspiration supports blast pressure directly effecting the airway. This case has been well described in Military Medicine [8]. Searcy et al. describes a 34-year-old male casualty who suffered a blast injury complicated by sand aspiration. The patient reported facing the blast when it occurred. He arrived at our combat hospital with a Glasgow coma score of 15 and was hypotensive. Injuries included face, left flank, back, left lower extremity, and an open distal tibia and fibula fracture with a retained foreign body. After intubation in the emergency department, the patient was taken to the operating room for external fixation and wound debridement. CT imaging of the chest (Figs. 8.4 through 8.8) showed foreign radiopaque material in the trachea and bronchi consistent with aspirated sand.

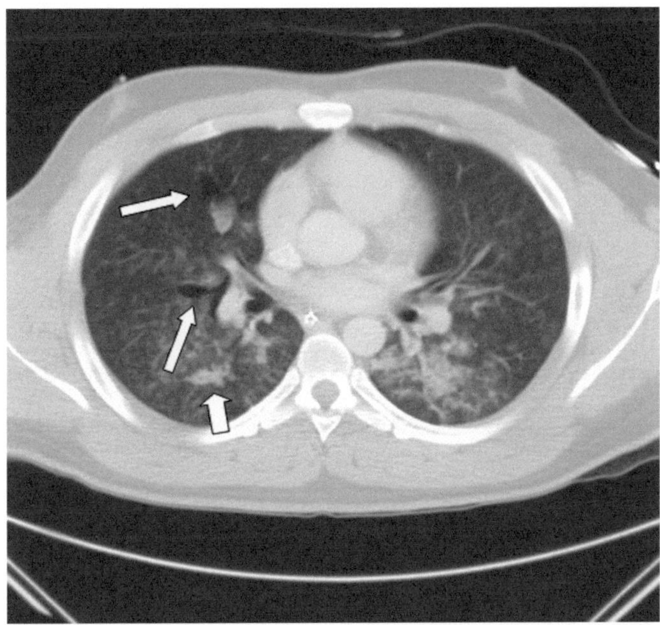

Fig. 8.2 Diffuse central consolidations and parenchymal tearing consistent with Blast Lung Injury from direct airway overpressure. Low attenuation areas represent focal lung parenchymal tearing (longer arrows). Focal patchy opacities seen here (shorter wide arrow) are essentially widespread pulmonary contusions and may have mixed components of edema/ARDS. Bronchial washings in the field in this case confirmed hemorrhage and blood components c/w diffuse contusions. Expiratory pressure waveform showed bleb-like flap effect

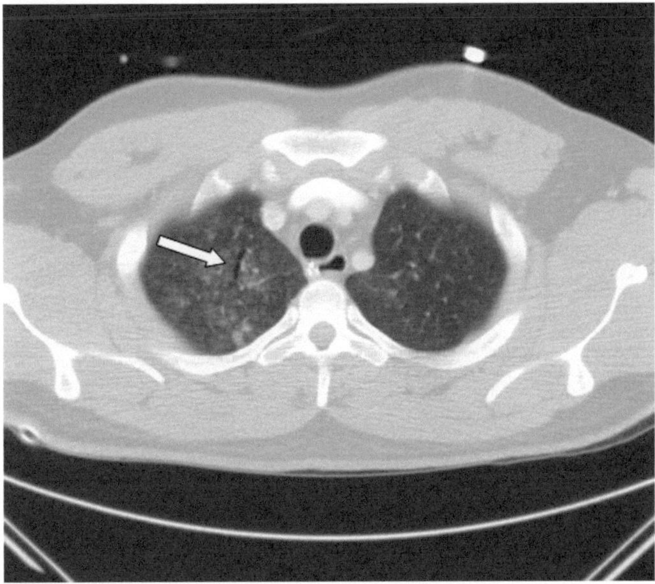

Fig. 8.3 Another lung parenchymal tear in the right apex (arrow)

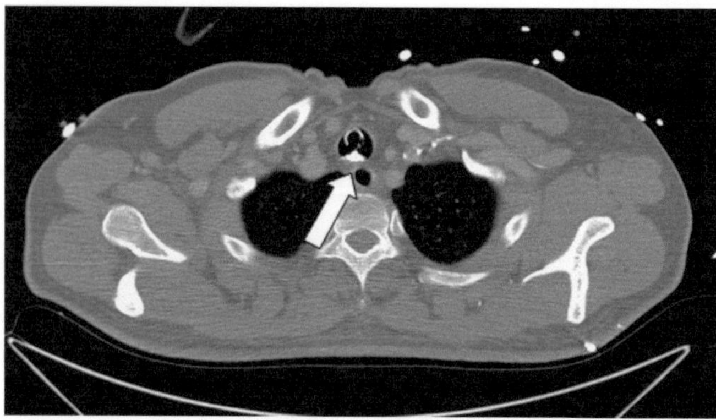

Fig. 8.4 Note the radiopaque material representing sand in the trachea (arrow) from a facial blast injury. Reprinted with permission from Military Medicine: International Journal of AMSUS

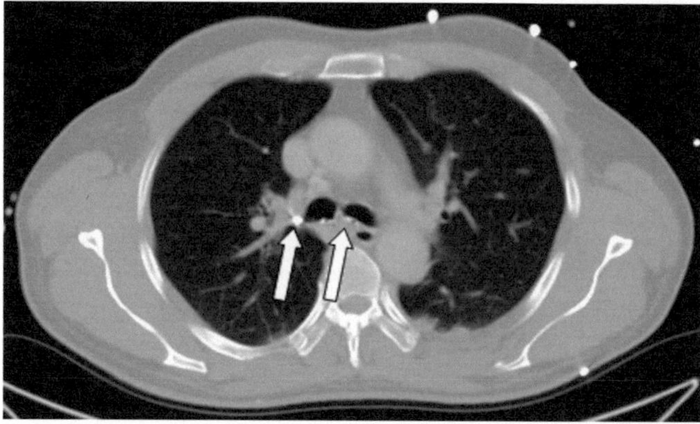

Fig. 8.5 Sand is noted right and left mainstem bronchi (arrows). Reprinted with permission from Military Medicine: International Journal of AMSUS

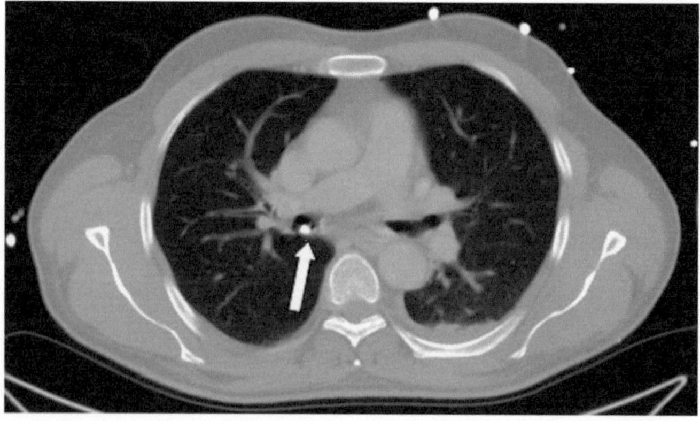

Fig. 8.6 Note the sand in a spherical shape in the right bronchus intermedius (arrow)

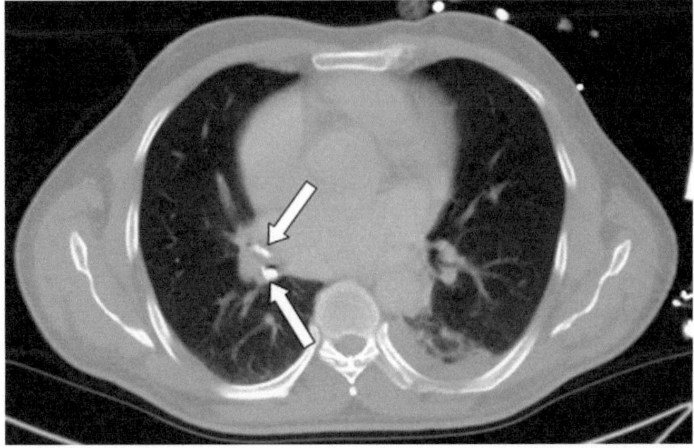

Fig. 8.7 Sand nearly obstructing the anterior and lateral basal bronchi segments of the right lung

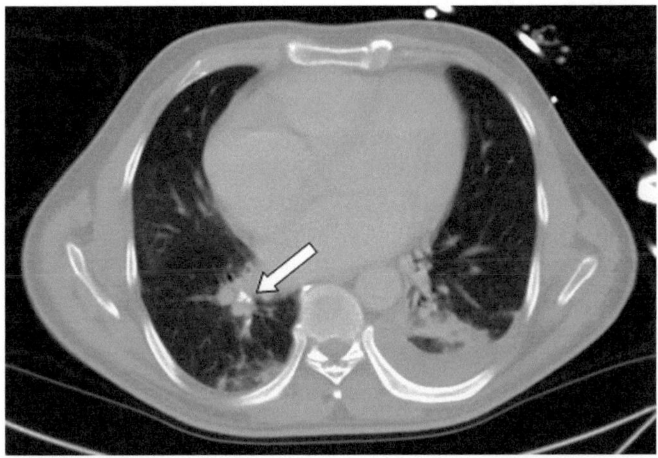

Fig. 8.8 Sand opacities were noted as far as the inferior portion of the posterior basal bronchi segment on the right. Note the left pleural effusion and basilar atelectasis

Following surgery, the patient was taken to the ICU and extubated. In the ICU, muddy secretions were suctioned from the respiratory tract, and bronchoscopy showed mild mucosal inflammation and yellow mud adherent to both the tracheal wall and the upper bronchi. Drowning following the blast was a consideration, until a more accurate history was obtained.

Sand aspiration is seen in drowning, direct inhalation, or blast injury. The CXR can support a diagnosis in cases of sand aspiration; however, CT is more sensitive. In a recent retrospective examination of postmortem CT (as opposed to conventional autopsy) in the diagnosis of drowning victims, sand and sediment in the bronchial tree were visualized by CT on nearly half of the drowning victims [9].

The first reported case of sand aspiration was in a drowning victim. There was report of difficult CPR due to obstruction of the oropharynx and mouth with sand [10]. Other reports have described sand aspiration such as cave-ins, drowning and near drowning, and sand castle collapse [11–15]. Sand aspiration can range from rapid death due to total occlusion of the airway and subsequent anoxic death to a spectrum of dyspnea, cough, and variable obstructive symptoms. An example presentation was in an MVA patient who aspirated sand and had significantly elevated peak airway pressure and difficulty with ventilation support [16].

Sand aspiration in casualties suffering from blast injury should alert clinicians to the airway mechanism of blast lung and careful monitoring for lung injury by CT and ventilation support parameters.

8.5.2 Generalized Overpressure/Compression

The next case demonstrates a generalized peripheral lung contusion demonstrated in Figs. 8.8 and 8.9 through Figs. 8.8–8.12. A detailed history and record of injury is worthy in this case. This casualty was a 21-year-old army sergeant who suffered an explosion while in a Hummvee (High Mobility Multipurpose Wheeled Vehicle). He arrived to the first hospital with a GCS 15, tachycardic, class 3 hemorrhage, normotensive, and temp 101.3. The initial CXR and pelvis images were without significant injury, there was no c-spine injury (nor tenderness), and patient went to the OR emergently for lower extremity injuries. He had massive soft tissue/skin loss to the

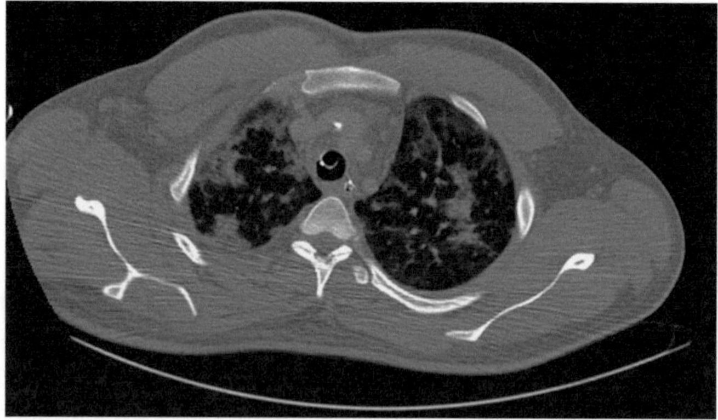

Fig. 8.9 Superior chest CT obtained immediately after this 21-year-old active duty Army soldier was in a confined space blast. Note the bilateral patchy consolidations distributed peripherally and centrally. The patient was intubated and had a central line and NG tube

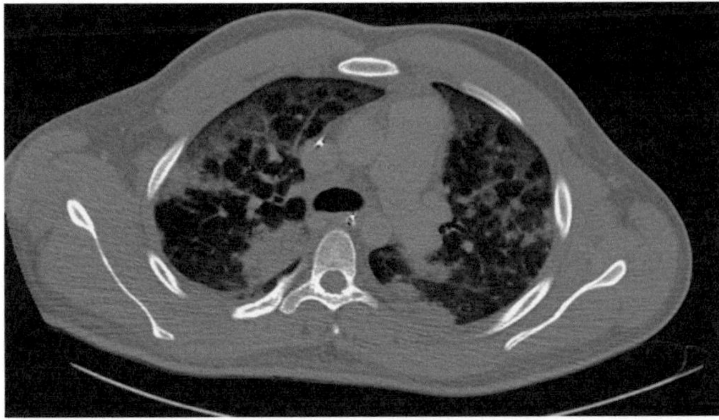

Fig. 8.10 A CT of the same casualty at the level of the carina showing the peripheral consolidations consistent with generalized blast overpressure contusion

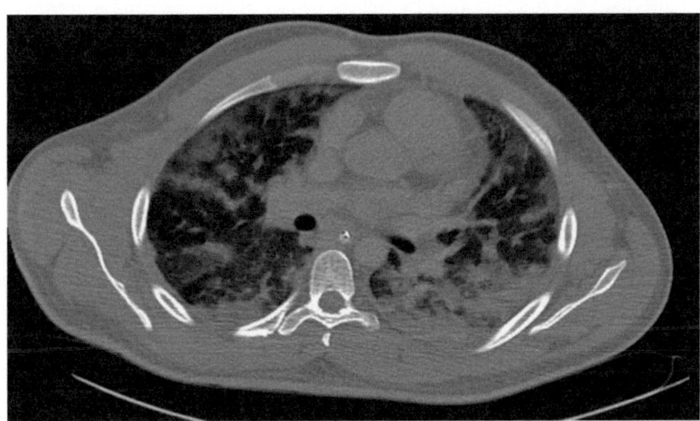

Fig. 8.11 This more inferior CT of the same blast patient shows slightly less peripheral contusion on the right, with increased contusion of the LLL posteriorly. There were more blast effects to the left side of his body, consistent with a more direct local lung hemorrhage to this area

right posterior thigh and leg, had right open foot fractures, left open knee, multiple fragment injuries to the upper and lower left leg. His left foot was mangled with near complete amputation of the leg at the level of the distal tibia. He was taken to surgery for where entire right leg had extensive hamstring and calf necrotic muscle, underwent a washout of right foot, washout of buttock wounds. He also had a complete amputation of the left foot above the ankle (distal tibia). After ET placement and right IJ central line, A-line, Foley catheter, had transfusion with two units packed red blood cells and four units fresh frozen plasma, then transferred to our hospital by helicopter.

On closer inspection at our hospital, he had bilateral acoustic trauma from blast, the patient was in shock with acute lung injury, requiring >70% FiO2 to maintain

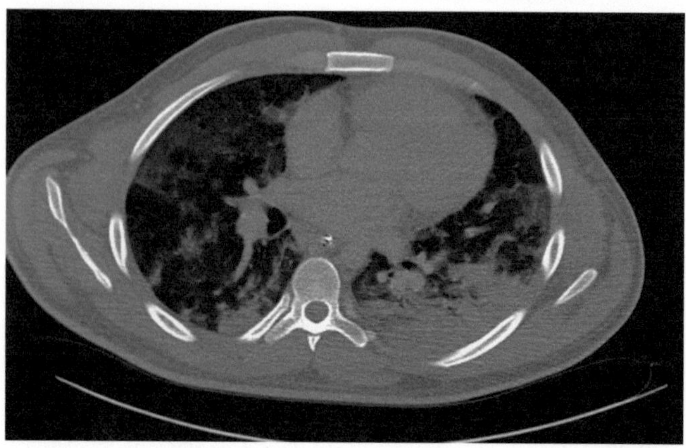

Fig. 8.12 The LLL typical contact contusion is noted in this image with air-bronchograms, note the right peripheral BLI pattern that has almost a mosaic or crazy paving type of distribution. This is thought to be due to the external forces of the thoracic cavity, as opposed to the more central type of blast injury patterns. This is supported by the inclusion of localized lung contusion from direct impact, and the peripheral airspace distribution

sats over 92%. CXR and CT showed bilateral diffuse airspace consolidations consistent with blast lung injury (Figs. 8.9–8.12). He had continued respiratory challenges in our hospital and in the air evacuation to Landstuhl Army Medical Center in Germany. There he also had CXR findings of BLI. One limitation to diagnosing BLI on CXR or even CT is that the picture is often complicated by ARDS; however, the BLI imaging findings seem more extensive than in civilian settings of ARDS posttrauma.

8.5.3 Focal Blast Injury to Lung

The next case shows a lung contusion from a direct impact from blast from the side (Fig. 8.13). The localized retained blast fragments support the direction of the blast and correlate with the consolidation distribution. Looking at all blast injuries to the chest over time, correlating history, exposure, confined space, distance, type of explosive and radiologic findings will help further define BLI, contusions, morbidity, and mortality of chest injuries and response to blast.

The following case is another example of focal lung injury resulting in contusion and highlights other radiographic features sometimes seen in blast injury worthy of review, to include hydropneumothorax. A casualty suffered an IED blast to the outside of his Hummvee. This 20-year-old soldier was in the passenger seat when the blast impacted the door resulting in an impact-type injury. See Figs. 8.14 and

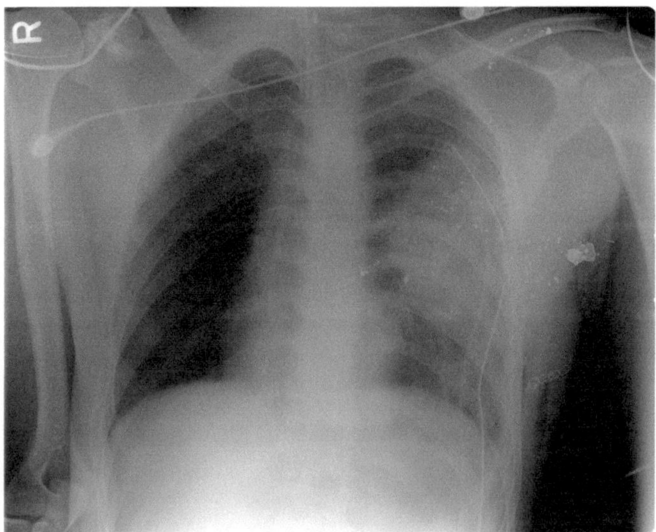

Fig. 8.13 Lung contusion from a direct blow from a blast from the left side. Note multiple retained fragments, subcutaneous air in the soft tissues, large airspace consolidation in the mid lung. The patient is intubated with an NG tube is satisfactory location. This is an example of a focal blast injury to the lung

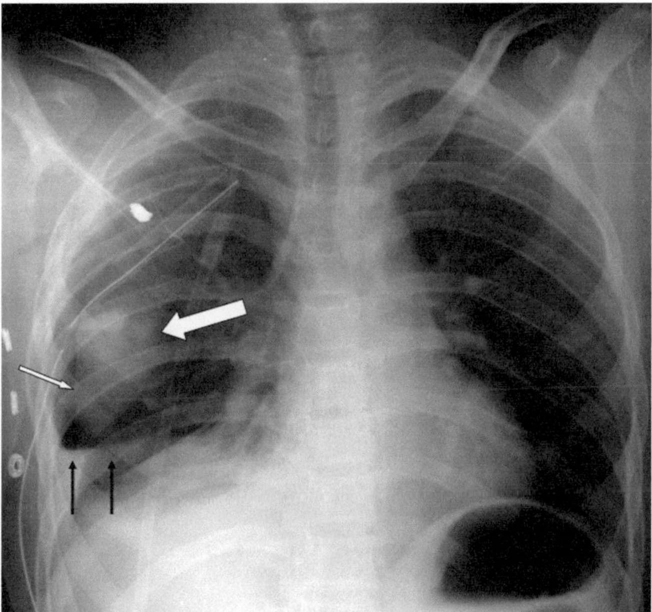

Fig. 8.14 Upright CXR showing the typical strait fluid level from a hemopneumothorax (black arrows). The pneumothorax is noted with the edge of the lung easily seen thin white arrow) in the region of the contusion (large white arrow). The chest tube is in satisfactory position. The blast fragment is noted overlying the upper right lung field

Fig. 8.15 A slightly oblique CXR demonstrating the blast fragment is actually just outside the lung and ribs. In locations where CT is not available, plain radiography can help triage by using traditional projections

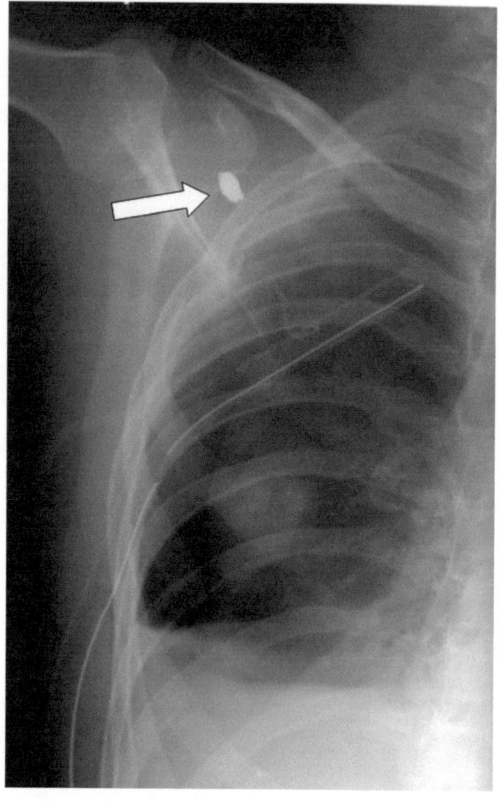

8.15 for upright CXRs showing the hemopneumothorax, blast fragment, and lung contusion from impact from the door. A good review of hydropneumothorax verses the meniscus sign seen in pleural effusion compared with teaching models is available [17].

The following child was the victim of a firefight as a bystander at a distance. This AK-47 round penetrated the left chest wall with low energy and ended up in the left pleural space. Fig. 8.16 shows the bullet overlying the left upper abdomen (as well overlying the lower lung) and Fig. 8.17 demonstrating the bullet in the sulcus of the lung. Note the two different locations of the bullet in this child. This demonstrates how inferior the lung sulcus projects. Note the lung contusion from the impact of the GSW.

This next case highlights (Fig. 8.18) how the CXR "scout" can help in the immediate follow-on care in the ICU. This patient was shot in the face with the bullet ending up in the trachea and has been well described by Cassleman [18]. After perforating the right mandible, the bullet missed major vasculature and penetrated the trachea. In Fig. 8.19, one can appreciate the location of the missile next to the ET tube. The patient had follow-up chest X-rays in the ICU showing progressive

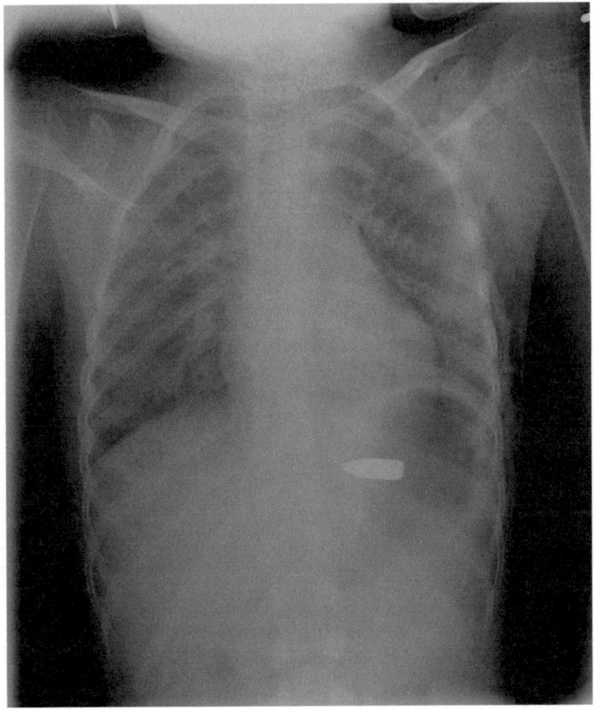

Fig. 8.16 The bullet is seen overlying the left upper abdomen, CT (not shown) demonstrated the bullet in the posterior (dependent) pleural space inside of a small pneumothorax

atelectasis, Figs. 8.20, 8.21, and 8.22. Consequently, urgent bronchoscopy performed shortly afterwards revealed the presence of blood in the patient's airway, completely obstructing his right mainstem bronchus. The patient improved dramatically and the last CXR showed markedly improved aeration of the right lung, not dissimilar to recovery after a mainstem intubation correction.

8.6 Summary

Chest imaging is diagnostic radiology at its best. Chest CT is our visual biopsy of the chest and provides definitive anatomic/pathologic process description to the trauma surgeons and ICU staff. Chest X-ray rounds are the important start to the combat hospital daily routine. In my opinion, they are the pulse of the battlefield hospital and indicator of clinical status. They also provide radiologists with clinical

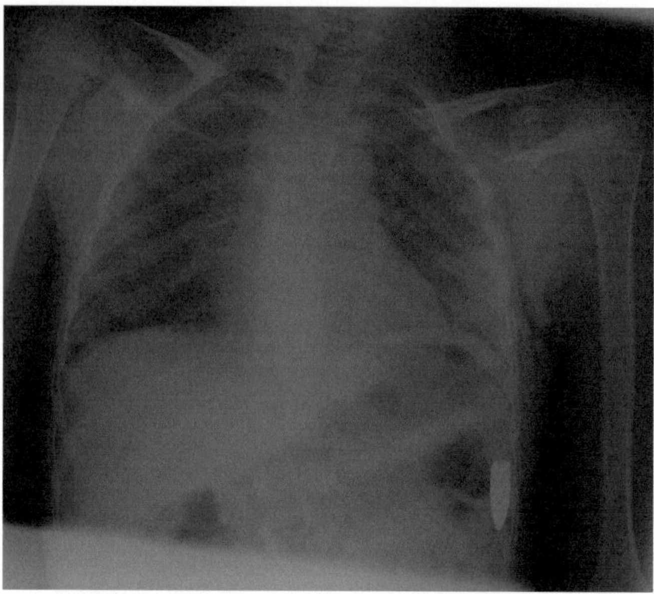

Fig. 8.17 The next day the bullet had migrated inferiorly and laterally as the child was sitting up and walking around. The dependent motion over time supports the location in the pleural space; this also shows how inferiorly the pleural sulcus projects and can appear as if in the abdomen

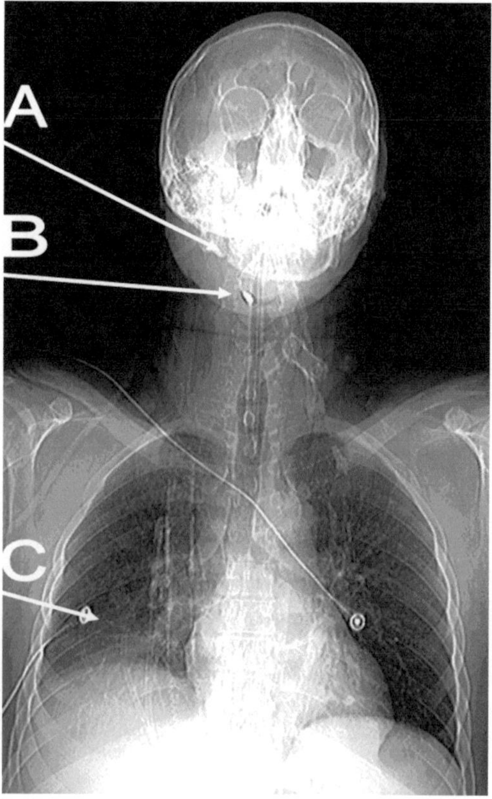

Fig. 8.18 CT scout of head, neck, and chest of GSW patient. Note fracture of mandible (A), bullet (B), and developing RLL atelectasis (C). Reprinted with permission from Military Medicine: International Journal of AMSUS

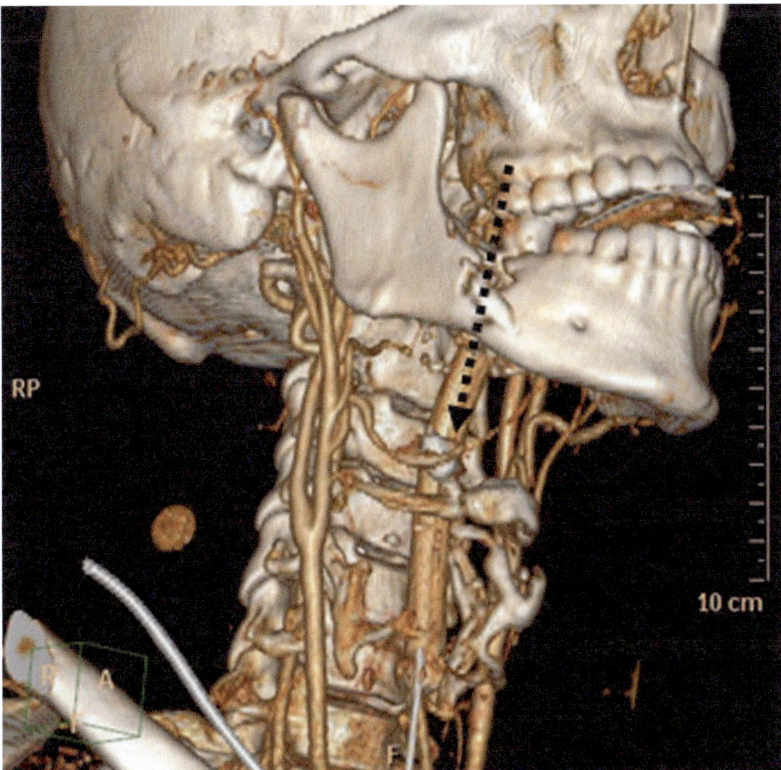

Fig. 8.19 A 3D volume rendered image showing the mandible fracture from the bullet and the proposed trajectory of the bullet (dotted arrow). The bullet ended up in the trachea next to the ET tube

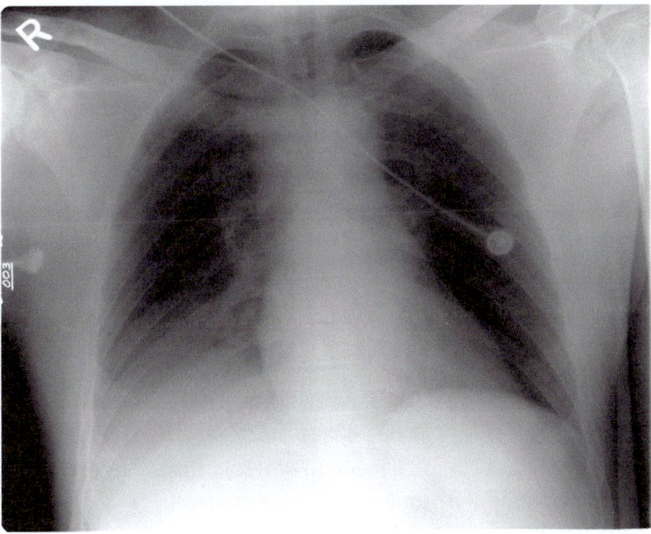

Fig. 8.20 A few hours after transfer to ICU, the RLL atelectasis was developing. A repeat CXR was recommended after a few hours to rule out major airway obstruction. Reprinted with permission from Military Medicine: International Journal of AMSUS

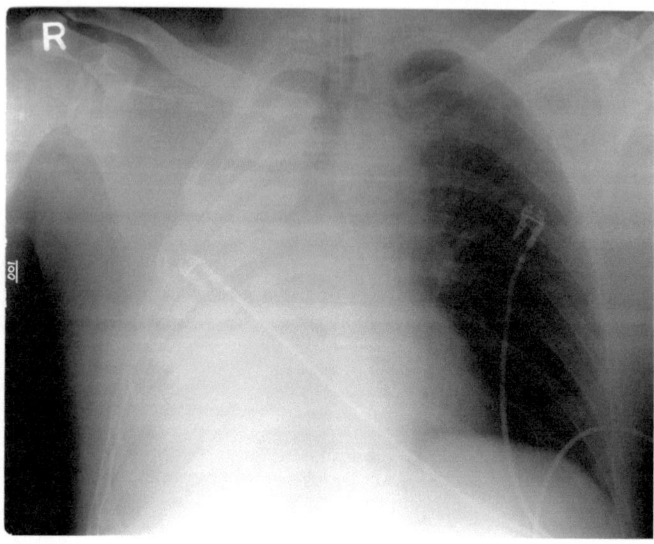

Fig. 8.21 Several hours after the injury near-total collapse of the right lung was noted. An urgent brochoscopy was recommended. Reprinted with permission from Military Medicine: International Journal of AMSUS

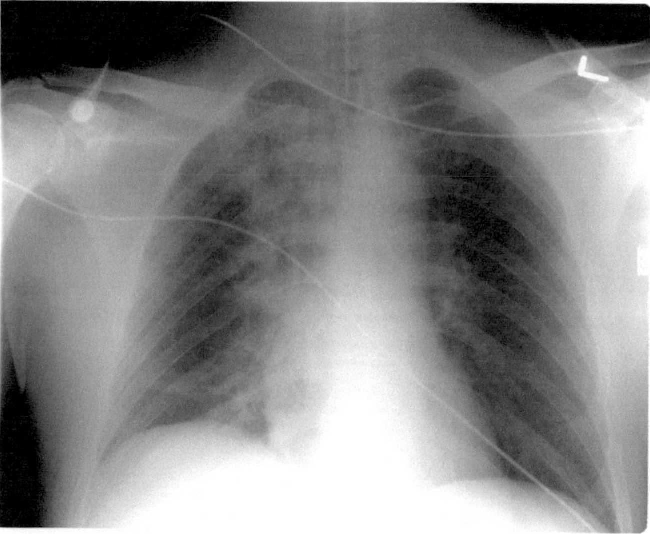

Fig. 8.22 Improved aeration of the right lung following urgent bronchoscopy. Reprinted with permission from Military Medicine: International Journal of AMSUS

information that may help provide a more useful and timely interpretation. Further, immediate interaction and interpretation may prevent unnecessary chest CTs for the less experienced to get a better feeling for what is going on. In my opinion, the common CXR provides more information than many may think, the CT has often been obtained to confirm what information already exists on the CXR.

I mentioned early in this chapter about the pace and stress of being a radiologist in combat. However, I am periodically reminded in private practice jobs, even today, that being a radiologist is a fast-paced profession everywhere. The major differences are that our lives were threatened on a regular basis, being attacked every day, the injuries were horrific, and the tent environment was challenging. Other than that, we are radiologists and busy wherever we are – this is a good thing.

References

1. Waninger KN, Rothman M, Foley J, Heller M. Computed Tomography is Diagnostic in the Cervical Imaging of Helmeted Football Players With Shoulder Pads. J Athl Train. 2004,39 (3):217–22.
2. DePalma RG, Burris DG, Champion HR, Hodgson MJ. Blast injuries. N Engl J Med. 2005 Mar 31,352(13):1335–42.
3. Coppel DL. Blast injuries of the lungs. Br J Surg. 1976 Oct,63(10):735–7.
4. Hare SS, Goddard I, Ward P, Naraghi A, Dick EA. The radiological management of bomb blast injury. Clin Radiol. 2007 Jan,62(1):1–9.
5. Wagner RB, Crawford WO Jr, Schimpf PP. Classification of parenchymal injuries of the lung. Radiology. 1988,167:77–82.
6. Avidan V, Hersch M, Armon Y, et.al. Blast lung injury: clinical manifestations, treatment, and outcome. Am J Surg. (2005),190:927–31.
7. Schnyder P, Wintermark M. Radiology of blunt trauma of the chest. Berlin, Springer, 2000.
8. Searcey BK, Jackson AM, Folio L. Facial Blast Injury Resulting in Sand Aspiration. Mil Med. 2009 Jan,174(1):23–4.
9. Levy AD, Harcke HT, Getz JM, Mallak CT, Caruso JL, Pearse L, Frazier AA, Galvin JR. Virtual autopsy: two- and three-dimensional multidetector CT findings in drowning with autopsy comparison. Radiology. 2007 Jun,243(3):862–8.
10. Hewer CL. Drowning. Lancet. 1962,1:636.
11. Dunagan DP, Cox JE, Chang MC, Haponik EF. Sand aspiration with near-drowning. Radiographic and bronchoscopic findings. Am J Respir Crit Care Med. 1997 Jul,156(1):292–5.
12. Efron PA, Beierle EA. Pediatric sand aspiration: case report and literature review. Pediatr Surg Int. 2003 Jul,19(5):409–12. Epub 2003 Jun 11.
13. Bender EM, Moore EE, Kashuk JL, Hopeman AR. Conservative management of sand aspiration: case report. Mil Med. 1984 Feb,149(2):98–9.
14. Wales J, Jackimczyk K, Rosen P. Aspiration following a cave-in. Ann Emerg Med. 1983 12:99–1.
15. Glinjongol C, Kiatchaipipat S, Thepcharoenniran S. Severe sand aspiration: a case report with complete recovery. J Med Assoc Thai. 2004 Jul,87(7):825–8.
16. Dunagan DP, Cox JE, Chang MC, Haponik EF. Sand aspiration with near-drowning. Radiographic and bronchoscopic findings. Am J Respir Crit Care Med. 1997 Jul,156(1):292–5.
17. Reed A, Dent M, Lewis S, Shogan P, Folio L. Hydropneumothorax. Mil Med. 2010 Aug, 175(08).
18. Cassleman J, Zakaroff M, Folio L. Progressive atelectasis secondary to GSW to airway.Mil Med. 2009 May,174(5): 2 xvii–xviii.

Chapter 9
Abdomen and Pelvis Imaging in Iraq

Keywords Temporary abdominal closure (Balad Pack) · VII systemic clotting agents · Quick-clot®

9.1 Introduction

The majority of the injuries during the time I was in Iraq were blast and ballistic injuries; this was especially true for the abdomen and pelvis due to lack of body armor in these regions. Like any other trauma center, the pelvis AP X-ray was second only to the CXR. The plain X-rays of the abdomen and pelvis were often used as a survey of retained blast fragments and major fractures.

In the ICUs and wards, abdomen images could evaluate for ileus, obstruction from surgery or other complications, feeding or NG tube placements, stone protocols, or infections. I will show cases that are more unique to combat injury applications.

9.2 Cases

I would like to start off with a case highlighting an abdominal condition that is seen on CXR indirectly with an unusual finding: a chest tube coming from the abdomen and a vascular surgical clamp that was left in the belly to stop a major vascular bleed of the liver, not an unusual site in combat hospitals. See Fig. 9.1 for a wounded warrior shot in the abdomen with a high-velocity weapon that transferred much of its energy to the liver, resulting in major laceration. See Figs. 9.2 and 9.3 for operative photos of the liver during surgery, and Fig. 9.5 for the abdominal closure dressing that was used daily in our combat hospital. Clamps were placed prior to a right partial hepatectomy to control bleeding and left in place during the temporary abdominal closure (what we call "Balad pack" at the AF theater hospital). This ICU patient underwent damage control surgery before CT could be performed. The hemostat is actually clamping the liver across the right lobe

L. Folio (ed.), *Combat Radiology: Diagnostic Imaging of Blast and Ballistic Injuries*,   171
DOI 10.1007/978-1-4419-5854-9_9, © Springer Science+Business Media, LLC 2010

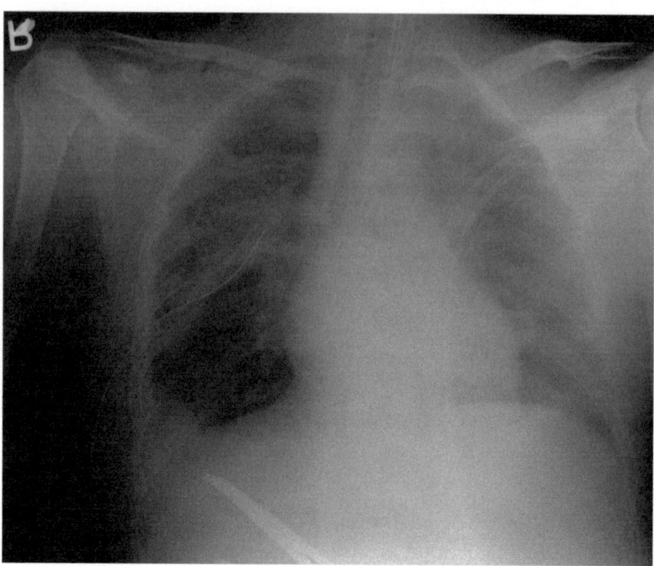

Fig. 9.1 Note the hemostat overlying the RUQ. Overlying instrumentation is taken into different consideration in combat imaging. It is not uncommon to have surgical sponges, hemostats, and other equipment remaining in the patient after initial damage control surgery. The chest tube coming from the abdomen in the center is entering the abdomen incision covered by an abdominal closure that covers the abdomen after immediate surgery, to allow for re-entry for surgical follow-up after initial stabilization. The clamp in the RUQ is actually in the abdomen as it remained within the Balad pack (see Fig. 9.5). There is a faint deep sulcus sign from a right anterior-inferior pneumothorax, with an airspace opacity in the RLL representing lung contusion

vascular pedical to stop bleeding due to trauma. These creative life-saving measures have evolved from the challenges of combat medicine.

Large clamps were placed along the line of liver resection and remained in place following the initial operation. The abdomen was temporarily closed as part of his initial damage controloperation (Figs. 9.4 and 9.5). See Fig. 9.6 for more definitive closure.

See Fig. 9.7 for a coronal reformation of an example large soft tissue wound from a penetrating blast injury that was field treated with a clotting agent to stop the bleeding called Quick-clot®. Quick-clot® (Z-Medica Corporation, Wallingford, CT) [1] is a field clotting agent that is applied directly to large, open wounds [2]. It is very radiodense on X-ray and CT. The mud/ sand in Iraq is very dense and often appears as more radiodense than bone, less than metal (no beam hardening). Many other medical advances have helped save the lives of deployed troops such as a one-armed tourniquet and factor VII clotting agents [3].

The following case highlights some typical radiologic body findings in blast injury. The following patient (Figs. 9.8–9.14) had primary blast lung injury (see chapter on blast injury types) demonstrated by diffuse consolidates sometimes seen in mild blast lung (see chapter on chest, section on BLI), in addition had secondary and tertiary blast injury. See Chap. 3 for blast injury types, and Chap. 8

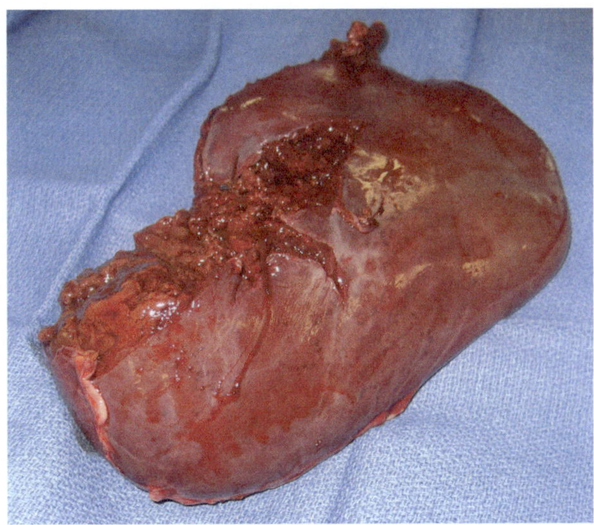

Fig. 9.2 This patient suffered a high-velocity GSW to the abdomen that penetrated the posterior right hepatic lobe and exited just to the left of Cantlie's line. Note the damaged liver section that was surgically removed when attempts at packing were unsuccessful during his initial damage control operation

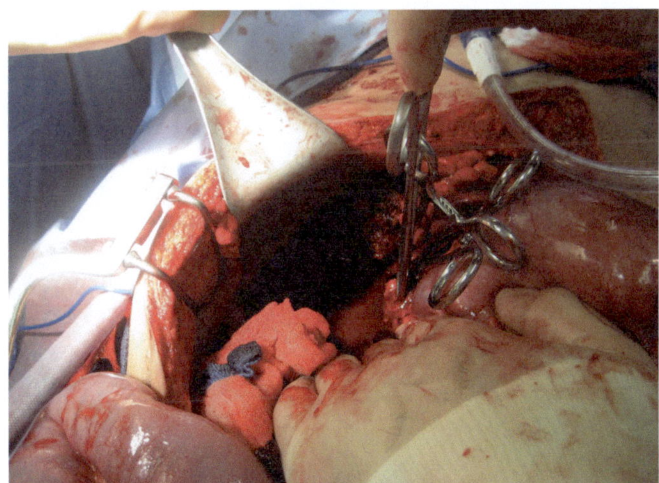

Fig. 9.3 Large clamps were placed along the line of liver resection and remained in place following the initial operation. The abdomen was temporarily closed as part of his initial damage control operation

for the three major radiologic manifestations of BLI. The patient also had a grade IV splenic laceration radiographically. There was fluid in the peritoneum: perisplenic, perihepatic, and pelvic. This case also demonstrates an excellent example of shock

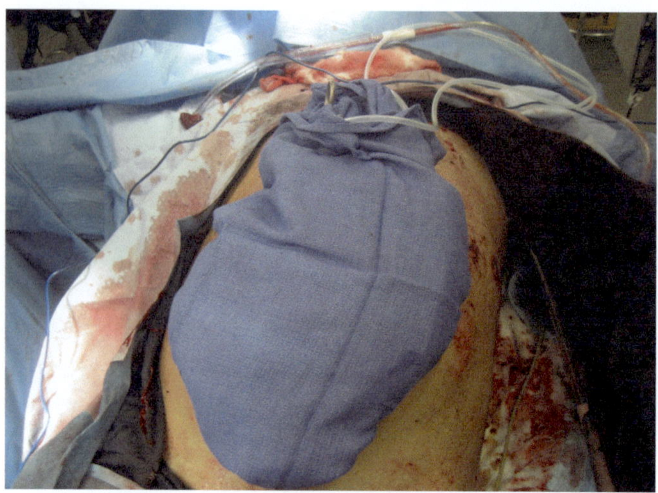

Fig. 9.4 The "Balad pack" can be seen covering the clamps, with the definitive closure photo shown last. Note the handles of the clamps just under the translucent pack superiorly. The clamps were removed prior to definitive abdominal closure

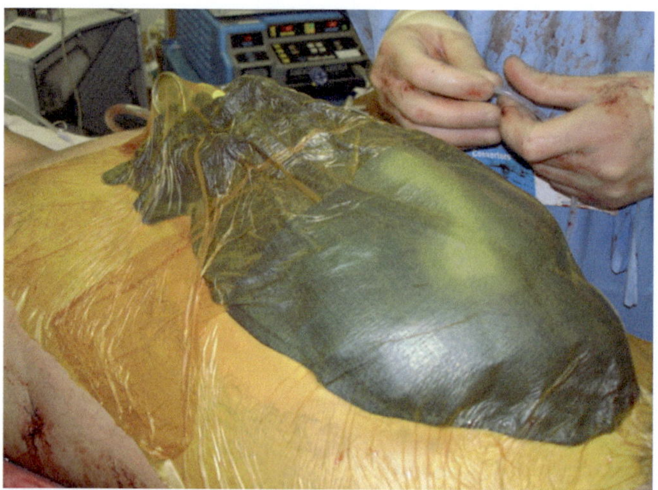

Fig. 9.5 The Balad pack seen here following the last step of plastic covering to seal the abdomen (with exception from the chest tube to prevent abdominal compartment syndrome.) Operative photos and caption descriptions courtesy of Matt Sena, MD, UC Davis Medical Center

bowel in an adult [4]. Shock bowel is not uncommon in blast injuries and makes sense from a mechanistic perspective. There were also fractures of rt 11th rib and most lumbar spine transverse processes. The bone fragments in the cecum are likely dietary and not an uncommon finding in patients seen in Iraq.

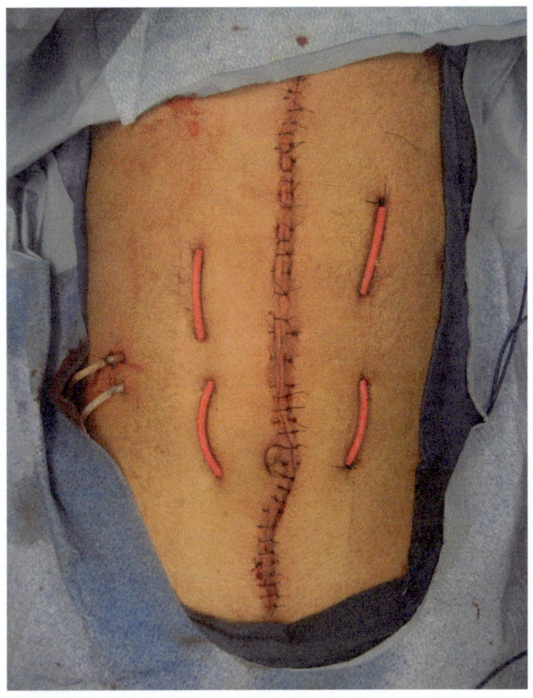

Fig. 9.6 Following definitive surgery, the abdomen is closed traditionally

The next case represents a blast injury from the seat of a vehicle (very common) that resulted in a severe lumbar spine body fracture with psoas hematoma with active bleeding, shock bowel, and flat, dense (with contrast) IVC. This casualty had active bleeding contrast blushing/extravisation of the left gluteus and surrounding soft tissues. Soft tissue active bleeding in this region can be catastrophic and needs immediate attention. See Figs. 9.15–9.17 for example CT axial scans of abdomen and pelvis.These findings correlated well with active bleeding of this area in the ER with rapid swelling.

This next casualty suffered a close range blast to the right gluteal region. Note the numerous metallic blast fragments distributed throughout the muscles and soft tissues of the right thigh and gluteal region. Some of the more superficial fragments were removed, however, most remain (Fig. 9.18).

The following casualty was hemodynamically unstable after a blast injury. Select images of a positive FAST exam done in the ER demonstrate enough fluid in Morrison Pouch (lucency/fluid between kidney and liver) to triage patient to the operating room and bypass CT (Figs. 9.19 and 9.20).

Commonly seen abdominal emergency cases seen in civilian centers that are not combat specific are not covered here. It is, however, worthy to mention a high incidence of certain common emergent Disease Non Battle Injury (DNBI) imaging findings. For example, because of the heat, dryness, wind, and exhausting schedules (12–18 h days) compounded by dehydration, we see an unusually high percentage

Fig. 9.7 Coronal reformat of large gluteal fragment track, with characteristic quick-clot opacity seen filling the gaping wound

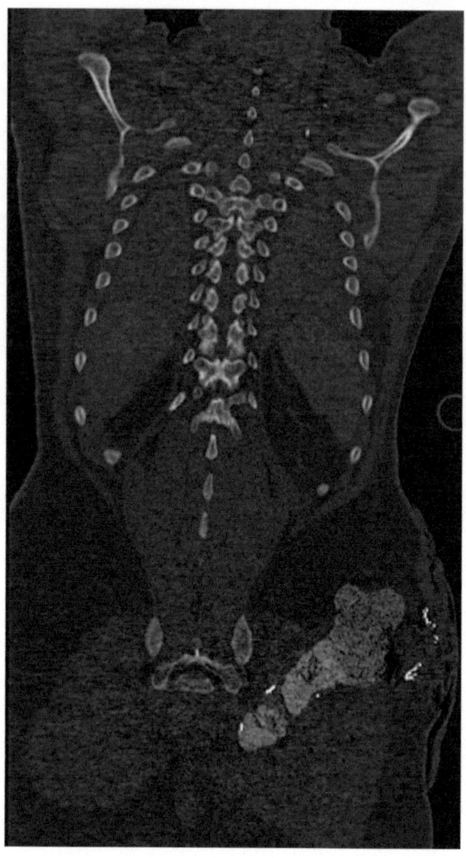

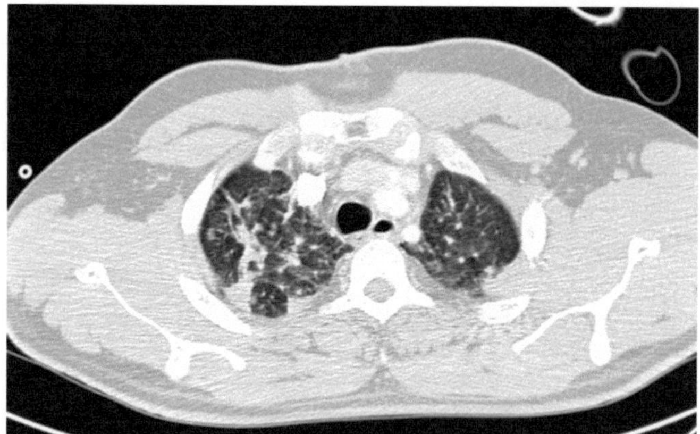

Fig. 9.8 CT of blast patient with generalized airspace opacities often seen in blast lung

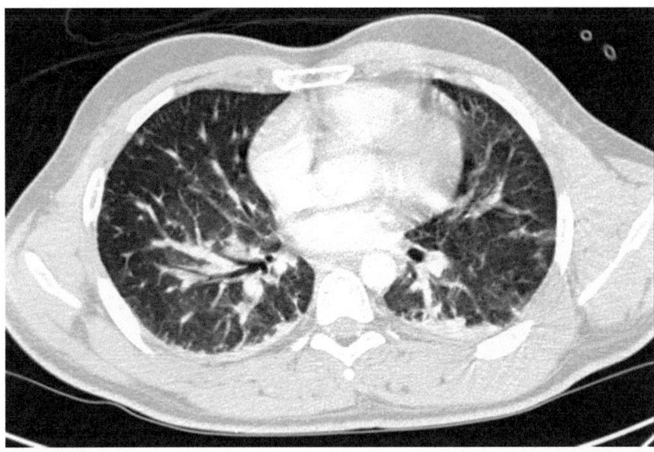

Fig. 9.9 Another chest CT showing diffuse airspace opacities centrally and peripherally

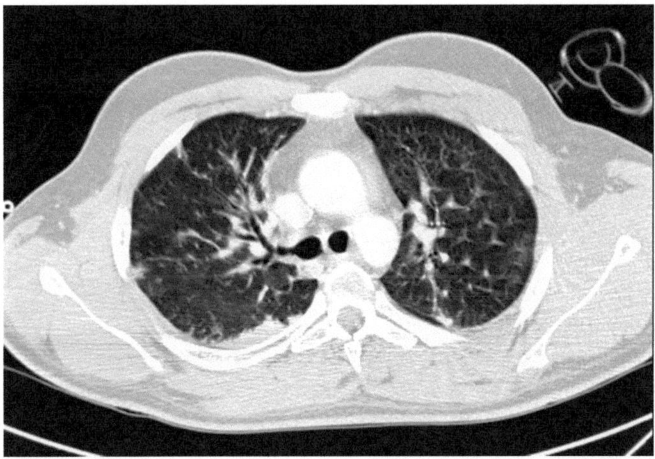

Fig. 9.10 A chest CT more inferiorly showing diffuse airspace opacities centrally and peripherally

of positive stone protocol CTs. These include ureteral lithiasis, resultant hydronephrosis, and hydroureter. Anecdotal experience and deployment patterns of urologic records reveal a probable correlation of stone diagnosis and incidence. Deployed radiologists and urologists agree on prior work that showed De novo synthesis of renal calculi development is likely approximately 93 days after arriving in the desert [5]. Our deployed urologist, Dr. Jeff Nelesnik provided antectodal data supporting these results for our deployment. Further research is needed in this area, taking seasonal variation, service specific (Army rotates differently than AF for example) variables into consideration.

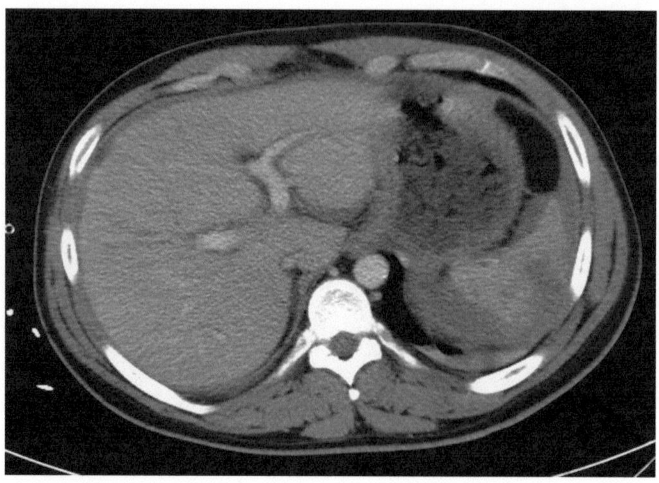

Fig. 9.11 Splenic laceration without evidence of active bleed, however, with perihepatic and perisplenic fluid

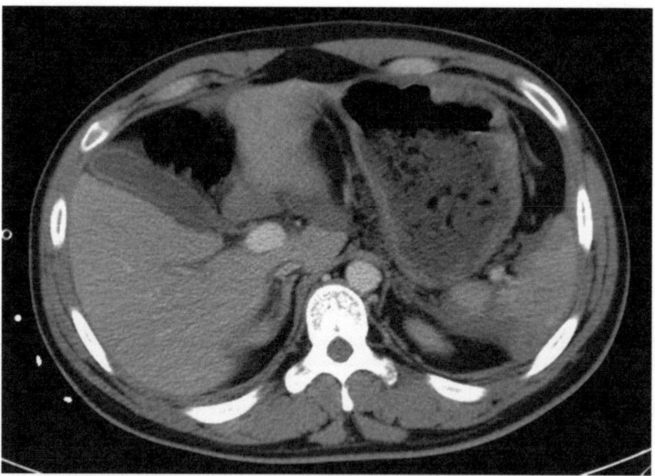

Fig. 9.12 CT at level of GB showing fluid around the GB and lacerated spleen

In our deployed hospital, we have a close working relationship with urology and have the flexibility to adjust the protocol based on findings. For example, if we cannot readily differentiate phelbolith versus a ureteric stone, we go ahead and give IV contrast without additional consultation to determine if there is indeed a stone. We also find it useful to mention whether or not any stones found on CT are seen on the scout view. This helps determine the makeup of the stone (taking size into

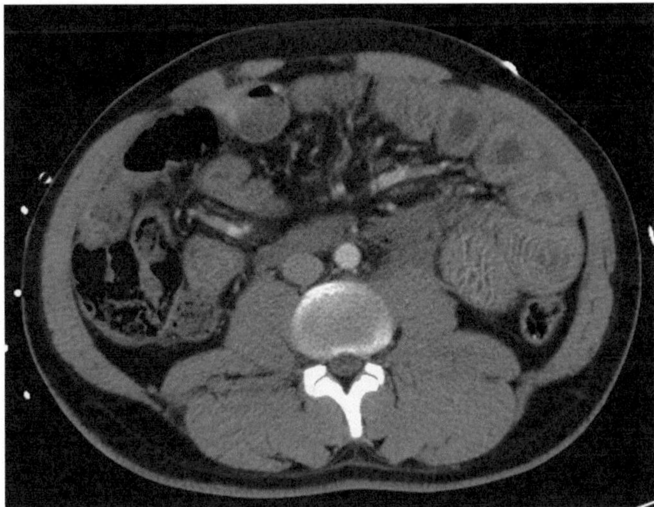

Fig. 9.13 Note the thickened, enhancing small bowel consistent with shock bowel. We often saw shock bowel without a flat IVC, due to aggressive IV hydration by the field medics and ED docs

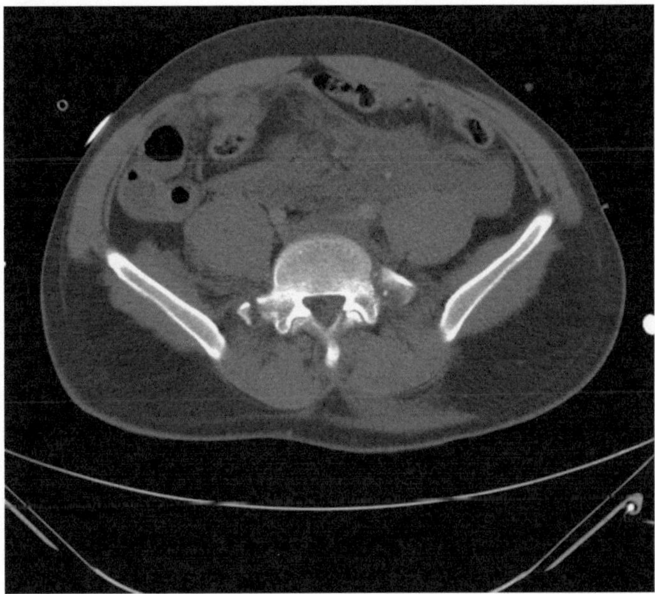

Fig. 9.14 Bilateral transverse process fractures of a transitional L5. These fractures were typical in patients exposed to blast, especially when in vehicles. One belief was that transverse process fractures were due to the heavy body armor and equipment worn on all field military at all times. The increased weight may have precipitated the transverse process fractures of the lumbar spine

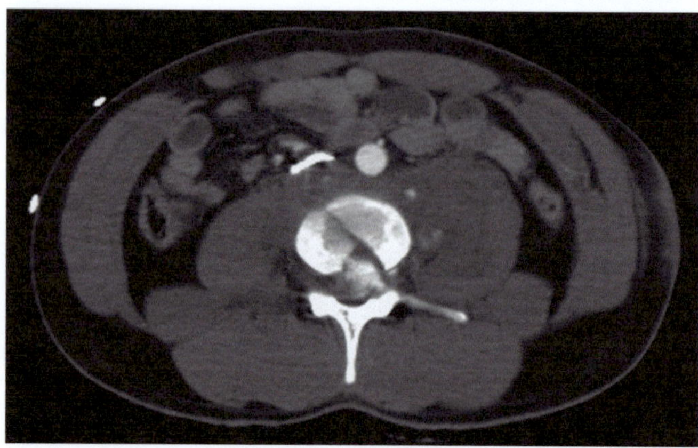

Fig. 9.15 Blast victim that sustained an L2 burst fracture with 90% canal compromise, with active bleeding and hematoma of left psoas muscle

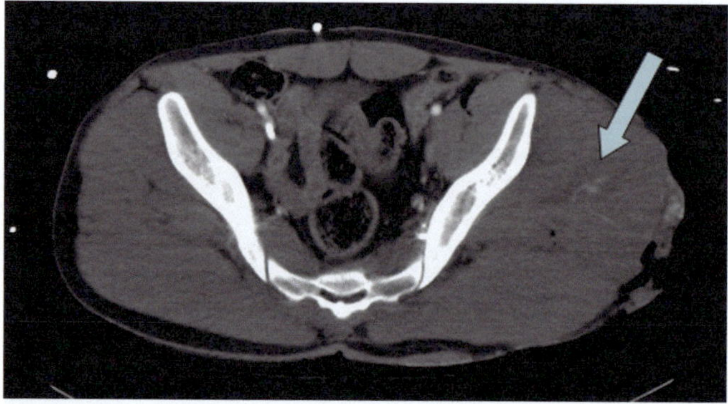

Fig. 9.16 There was also evidence of active contrast blushing/ extravasation of the left gluteus and surrounding soft tissues. This correlated well with active bleeding of this area in the ER. These injuries are not minor and need aggressive follow-up and potential embolization as one can lose a great deal of blood in this region

consideration as well) and is helpful for the urologist to guide therapy. Traditionally this is done with the KUB; however, further research may find the CT scout as an adequate analog for the KUB. There is potential that the digital processing of the scout may create some variation.

Emergent conditions not related to battle trauma are categorized under DNBI and are monitored by public health for health surveillance with seasonal and other periodic comparison. For example, the prevalence of appendicitis seems proportionally high, as well as testicular torsion. This could have been due to a younger population percentage of deployed troops. Our ultrasound machines are laptops with choice of transducers, color Doppler with duplex capability and of sufficient

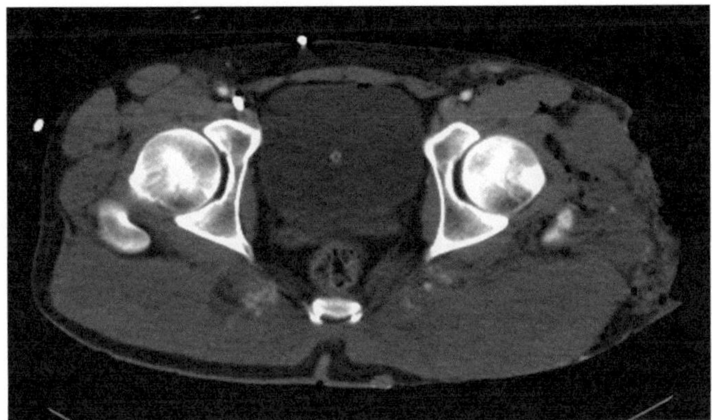

Fig. 9.17 Note the soft-tissue disruption to the left lateral thigh from the close proximity to the blast

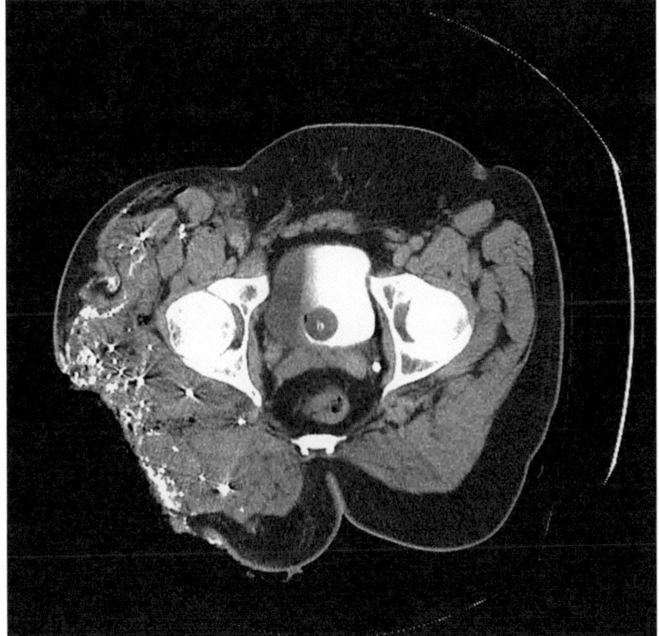

Fig. 9.18 Note the vast number of metallic fragments from this close proximity blast. This phenomenon is often called "peppering" presumably because of the clinical appearance as the debris is often dark from the explosive burning. Perhaps on CT we could call it "salting"

quality to detect testicular flow or lack thereof, to evaluate these as well as ovarian torsion. We were fortunate to have two ultrasound technologists. Other urgent ultrasound imaging diagnoses we could make include acute cholecystitis, DVT,

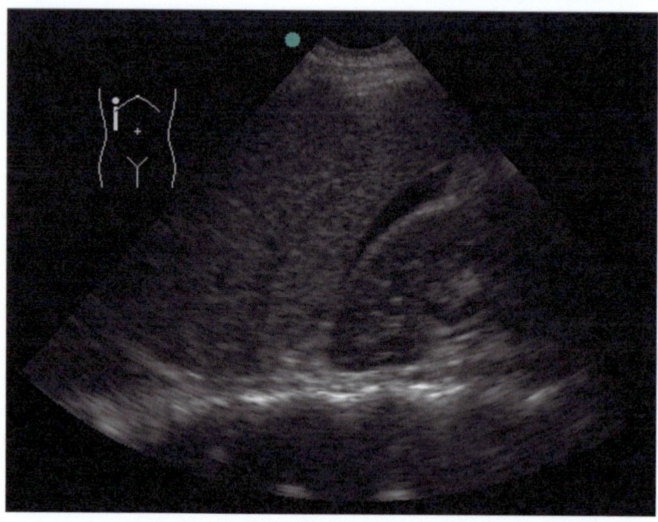

Fig. 9.19 Longitudinal FAST of the RUQ showing fluid in Morrison pouch

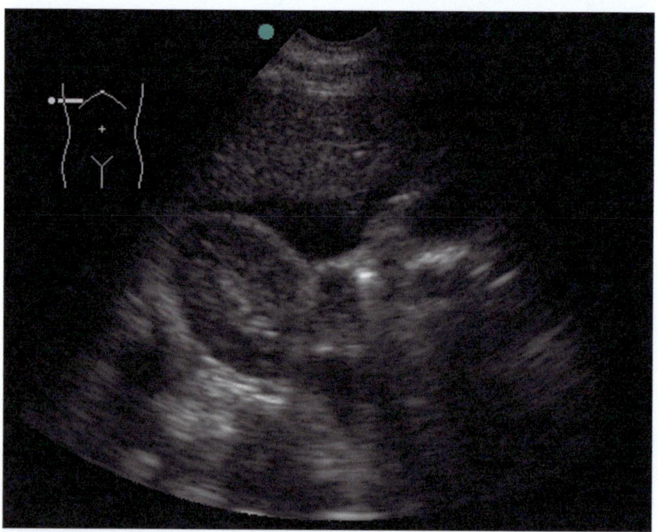

Fig. 9.20 Transverse FAST image of RUQ, supporting the free fluid in the abdomen

hernias, ovarian torsion, abscesses, Founiers gangrene, etc. Deployed radiologists are often asked to do intra-operative US for anatomical orientation or evaluation. It is not uncommon to be asked to assist in vascular access. The FAST and E-FAST US are mentioned elsewhere in this book.

9.3 Summary

Abdomen and pelvis injuries were common; however, with E-FAST and CT, we were able to guide surgeons to the most urgent cases and limit exploration surgically. Localizing fragments and, more importantly, analyzing the wound path for other organs damaged in the path was invaluable. Some cases are also available in the medical advances chapter where I discuss trajectory analysis of blast and ballistic injuries and Anatomic Positioning System for retained blast fragments.

References

1. Z-Medica Corporation, Wallingford, CT. http://www.z-medica.com/ (accessed Dec 09).
2. Ahuja N, Ostomel T, Rhee P, Stucky G et al. Testing of modified zeolite hemostatic dressing in a large animal model of lethal groin injury. J Trauma. 2006 Dec,61(6):1312–20.
3. Holcomb JB, McMullin NR, Pearse L, Caruso J, Wade CE, Oetjen-Gerdes L, Champion HR, Lawnick M, Farr W, Rodriguez S, Butler FK. Causes of death in U.S. special operations forces in the global war on terrorism: 2001–2004. Ann Surg. 2007 Jun,245(6):986–91.
4. Mirvis SE, Shanmuganathan K, Erb R. Diffuse small-bowel ischemia in hypotensive adults after blunt trauma (shock bowel): CT findings and clinical significance. AJR Am J Roentgenol. 1994 Dec,163(6):1375–9.
5. Evans K, Costabile RA. Time to development of symptomatic urinary calculi in a high risk environment. J Urol. 2005 Mar,173(3):858–61.

Chapter 10
Skeletal Trauma in Iraq

Keywords Morphing · External fixator · Missile embolus

10.1 Introduction

There are unique challenges to imaging extremities in a combat hospital environment and providing the information necessary to the orthopedic surgeons for surgical planning. Tremendous results have been witnessed in recent years with the judicious use of external fixators in the field [1]. In addition, wound vacuum-assisted closure along with aggressive forward field surgical approach, premier air-evacuation, and appropriate antibiotic therapy have helped limb salvage on the battlefield and in the higher echelons [2]. These temporizing stabilization and treatment modalities have saved the limbs of countless wounded warriors who would have otherwise lost their extremities or ended up with more severe disabilities such as those from prior conflicts. Example cases will be shown that have not been demonstrated in previous chapters, and only those unique to military combat setting. Again, even though military-specific from one perspective, any civilian setting can have combat-like conditions in a mass casualty disaster.

The first case demonstrates the potential horrific manifestations of blast/ballistics and burns/other wounds of combat (see Figs. 10.1 and 10.2). In addition to vascular concerns mentioned previously, extent of damage, degree of comminution, fragment location, and alignment are all important considerations.

See Figs. 10.3 and 10.4 for an unusual separation of the acromion from the scapula secondary to a bomb fragment perforating left shoulder. This case illustrates another advantage of 3D volume rendering, especially in complex orthopedic injuries. These help explain the nature of the injury to the surgeons, the commander, and other medical staff (Fig. 10.4).

L. Folio (ed.), *Combat Radiology: Diagnostic Imaging of Blast and Ballistic Injuries*,
DOI 10.1007/978-1-4419-5854-9_10, © Springer Science+Business Media, LLC 2010

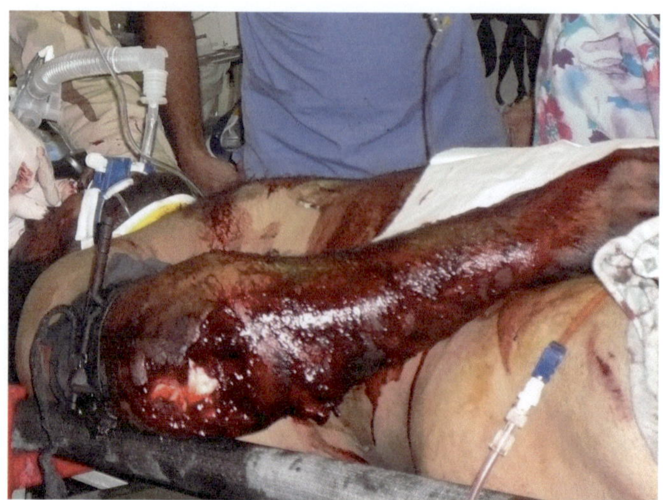

Fig. 10.1 This casualty was close to an IED blast and sustained a right lower leg amputation and fractures and fragments throughout other extremities and trunk

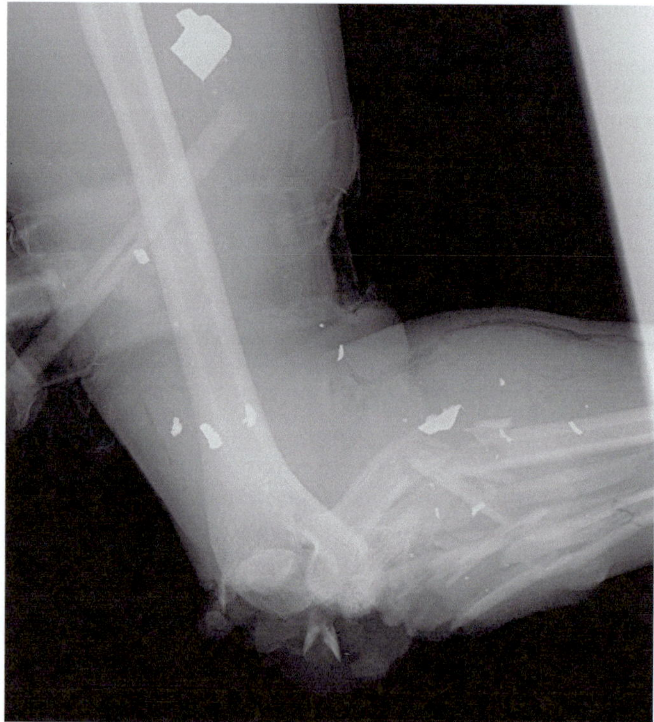

Fig. 10.2 Note the exposed right elbow on the X-ray showing the extent of soft tissue disruption. This correlates well with the photo

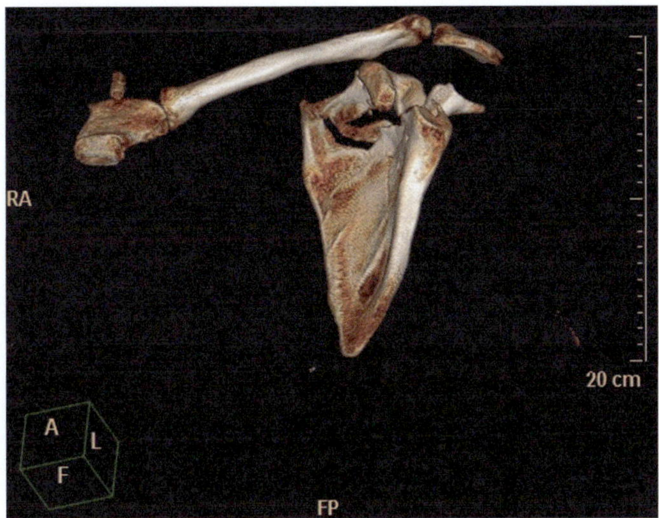

Fig. 10.3 3D view of scapular fracture with humerus subtracted to show extent of penetrating missile through acromion. Note the AC joint is maintained, however, the acromion is separated from the scapula from the projectile

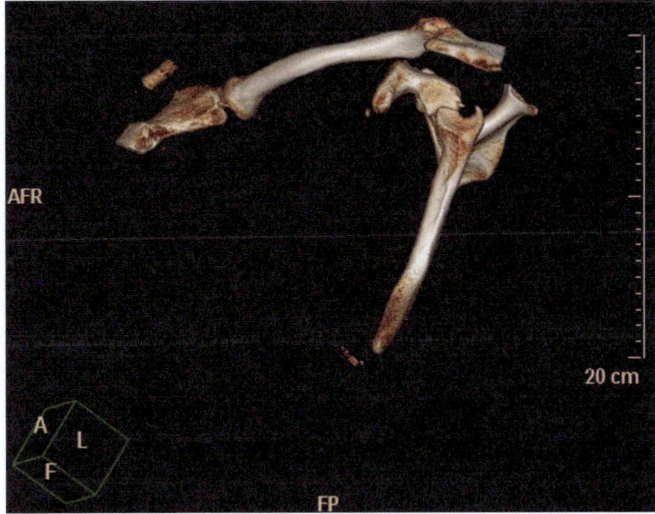

Fig. 10.4 Another perspective of the injury to show extent and relationships of fracture/separation

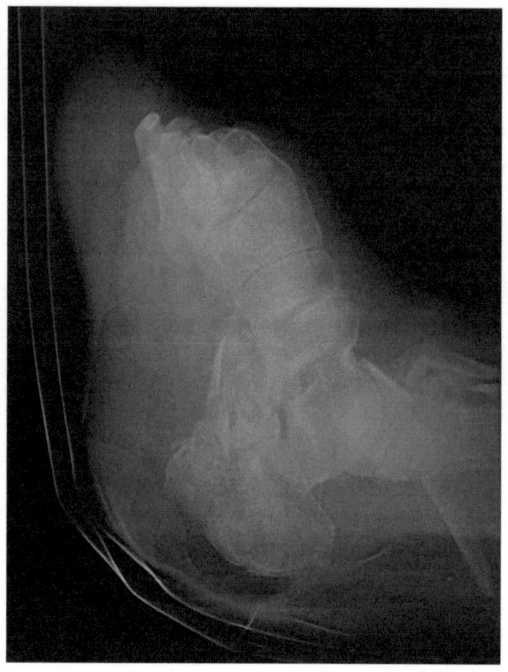

Fig. 10.5 This casualty had a prior exposure to blast resulting in a transmetatarsal amputation, back again for a severe comminuted and displaced tibia/fibular fracture to include severe calcaneous fracture. In addition to the prior trans-metatarsal amputation, note the severe impacted calcaneal fracture and marked soft tissue swelling inferiorly

Some of our patients arrived for second, third, or more visits. This made it challenging to differentiate new from old injuries. Many had retained blast fragments from prior blasts, and arrived at our hospital with a new blast with the possibility of new fragments. The Achilles Heel philosophy holds true in combat operations, as evidenced by the next few cases.

Figure 10.5 demonstrates a severe, impacted, and comminuted fracture of the calcaneous, as well as a severely displaced tibia/fibula fracture from a casualty with blast effects to lower extremities. This patient had a transmetatarsal amputation from a blast injury in the past. Unfortunately, the soft tissue and vascular integrity of this extremity were not sufficient to successfully salvage and resulted in a BKA (Figs. 10.6 and 10.7).

Calcaneal fractures can be complicated to treat for any individual or institution; however, compounding those fractures with associated soft tissue disruption makes treatment and rehabilitation or even limb salvage that much more challenging. For example, preservation of the soft tissues inferior and/or posterior to the calcaneous are important to salvageability of the foot. This next casualty had what may appear to be a simple soft tissue avulsion of the heel from a blast shearing injury, however, inclusion of the soft tissues and the bone made this difficult to salvage in this child (Fig. 10.8).

This last calcaneal fracture shown here is also severely comminuted, impacted and displaced, and compounded also by a displaced tibia fibula spiral fracture.

Fig. 10.6 This AP foot shows the prior trans-met with exostosis of the first metatarsal, soft tissue swelling and the calcaneal fracture displacement

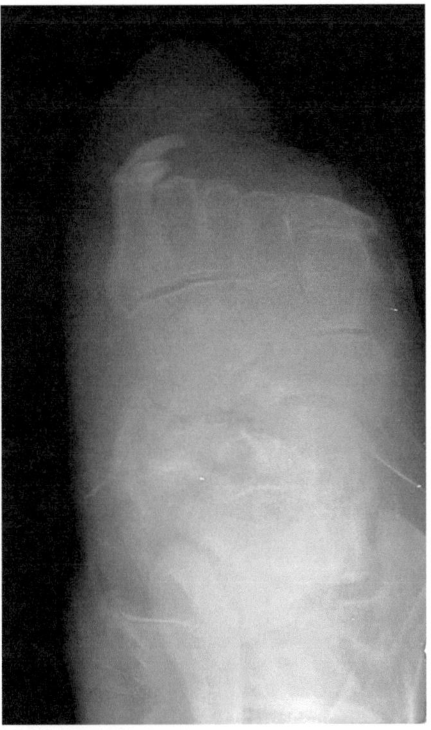

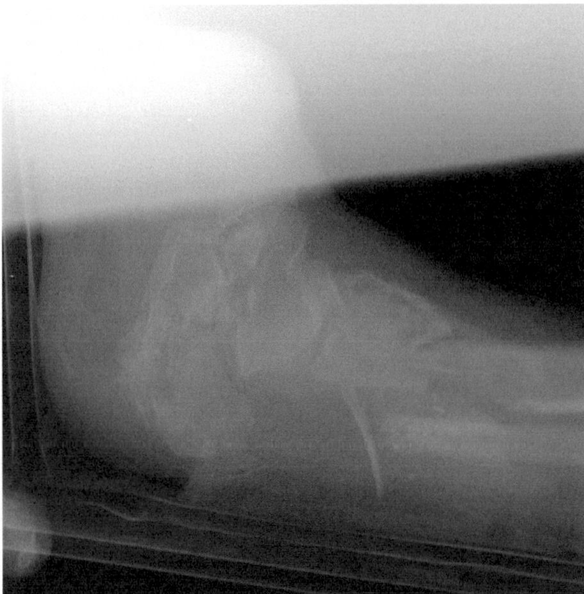

Fig. 10.7 To complicate potential limb salvageability in this returning war casualty, they also fractured their distal tibia and fibula with severe displacement and vascular and nerve damage

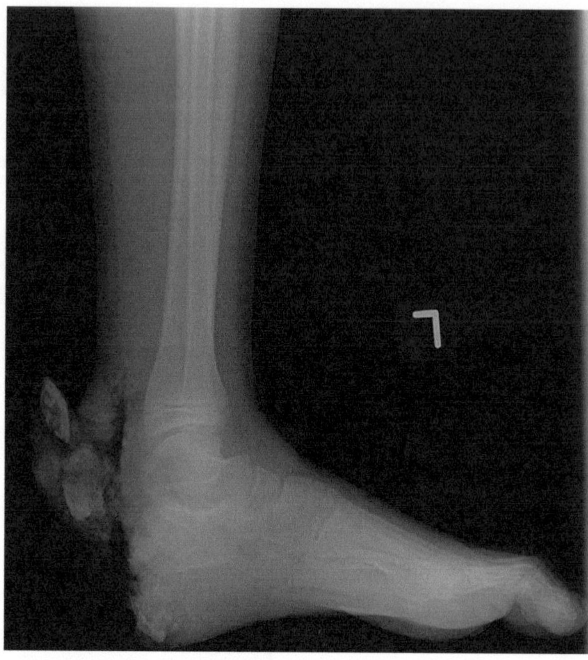

Fig. 10.8 This lateral X-ray of the foot and ankle demonstrates a major soft tissue avulsion from an explosion that also resulted in avulsion and communution of the calcaneous. One of the major predictors of clinical outcome in this case is the disrupted soft tissues of the heel, indicating a poor prognosis. Imaging may supplement the limb salvage prognosis, however, more research is needed in this area

Soft tissues were again disrupted, however, salvage, at least short term, was possible (Fig. 10.9).

If the AP and lateral extremity projections suggest metallic fragments in a joint space, exploration is likely in order, unless CT can help prevent surgery during busy times. Imaging can also determine whether or not a patient needs to be evacuated to Germany or the US for definitive care. The following case highlights this important role of imaging.

Although patella dislocations are not unique to military, there are certain considerations involving return to duty in combat that are unique, given the remote environment and austere conditions of the battlefield. The following describes a patient that dislocated his patella that was relocated in the ER without clinical complication. Our policy for returning soldiers to rigorous combat operations was to CT dislocated extremities to rule out avulsion fractures, loose bodies, etc. This helped in determining return to duty versus air-evacuation for definitive care and/or rehabilitation. It should be kept in mind that warriors deploy for up to over a year and may medical conditions cannot wait that long.

Fig. 10.9 Another example of disrupted soft tissues inferior to the calcaneous, with associated calcaneal fracture, along with spiral communuted intra-articular fracture of distal tibia

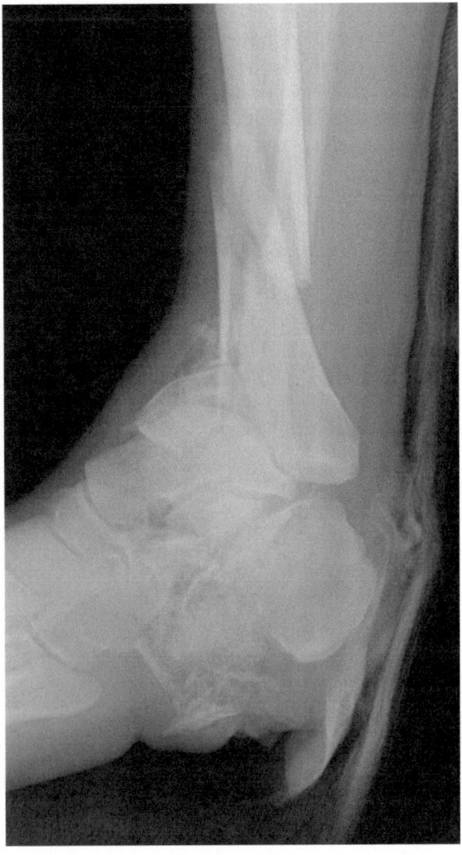

See Figs. 10.10 and 10.11 for a CT showing loose bodies in the patella bursa. Since this patient did suffer tiny avulsion fractures of the patella and femoral condyle articular surfaces, we recommended this soldier return to Landstuhl Regional Medical Center for scope and further evaluation (Figs. 10.12–10.14).

This unfortunate war casualty suffered an RPG (Rocket Powered Grenade) to the knee. In addition to severe comminuted, displaced fractures of the femur, tibia, and fibula, metal fragments and other debris resulted in horrific tissue damage. This injury resulted in extreme damage and an above the knee amputation was necessary.

Angiographic analysis of partial amputations and loss of skin can help determine salvageability of skin graft by identifying target vessels. Tissue flaps and free tissue transfer can be optimally determined with the help of CT and angiography, as well as limb salvage potential in theater (Fig. 10.15).

The next case demonstrates another penetrating injury to a joint. This artillery troop suffered a backfiring of a 50 caliber, the cap of the round projected from the

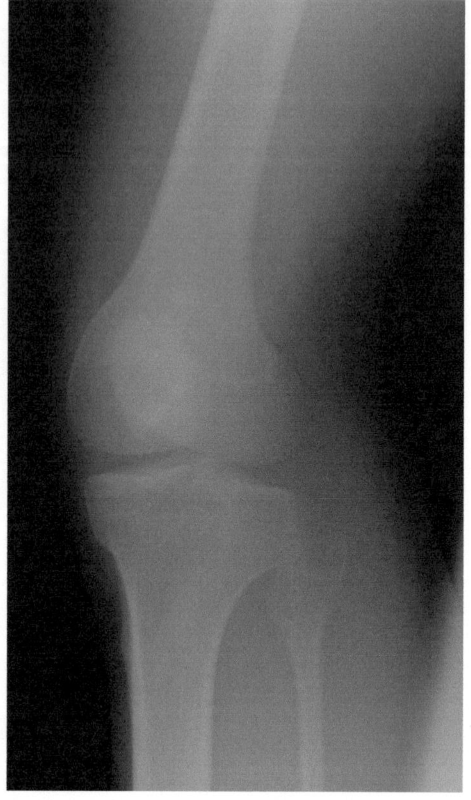

Fig. 10.10 AP knee of patella dislocation following first relocation attempt in field. The patella was dislocated laterally, definitively reduced in the ER and CT was done to rule our joint loose bodies since that influences management from an aeromedical standpoint

weapon and penetrated his elbow. The round section was removed without complication and patient was placed on antibiotics and returned to Landsthul Regional Medical Center for follow-up care and returned to theater in a few weeks.

The next case demonstrates embolization of a projectile to a pulmonary artery and is described by Andrews et al. [3]. See Figs. 10.16–10.18 for a 24-year-old helicopter navigator that was shot by an AK-47 round that penetrated his helicopter nose bubble before lodging in his left leg. A tourniquet was immediately placed on the navigator's thigh to control massive bleeding and then the helicopter diverted to a nearby combat support hospital within minutes. Surgical exploration and irrigation of his wounds occurred within 20 min of injury. Multiple metal and plastic fragments were removed from his leg. The X-ray of the knee showed a fragment in the popliteal fossa (among other fragments). The initial CXR was negative for fragments or other abnormality.

Five hours after injury, he became hypoxic and had increasing oxygen requirements. Follow-up chest X-ray demonstrated a new metallic fragment in the right lower lung field, vascular congestion, and mild hypoventilation. Another

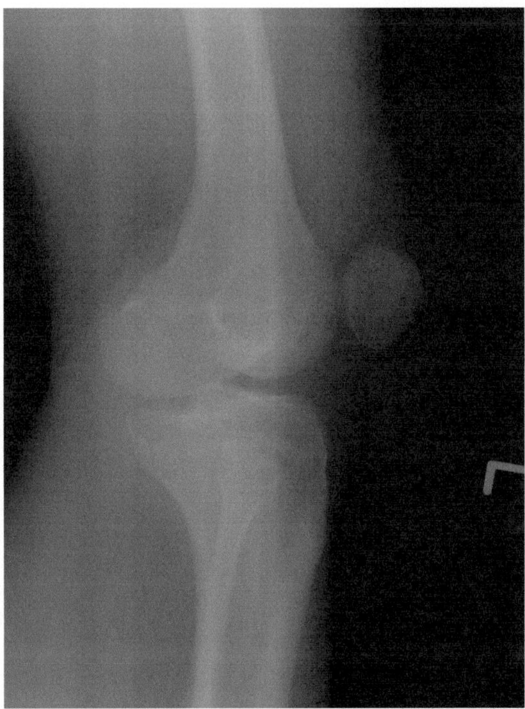

Fig. 10.11 Note the unusual appearance of the patella on the AP and slightly oblique portable lateral attempt in the ER

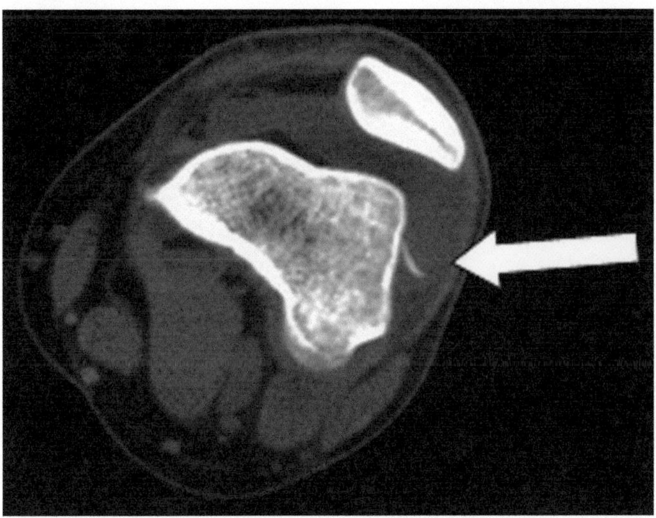

Fig. 10.12 CT demonstrated soft tissue swelling, joint effusion and several tiny avulsed bone fragments, this one of the lateral anterior femoral condyle (*arrow*)

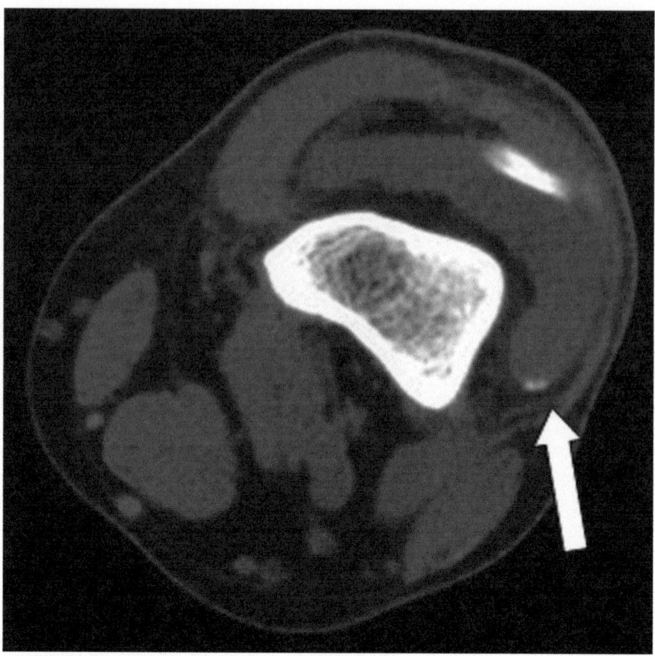

Fig. 10.13 Another CT demonstrating loose body fragments in the dependent (supine in CT) patella bursa (*arrow*)

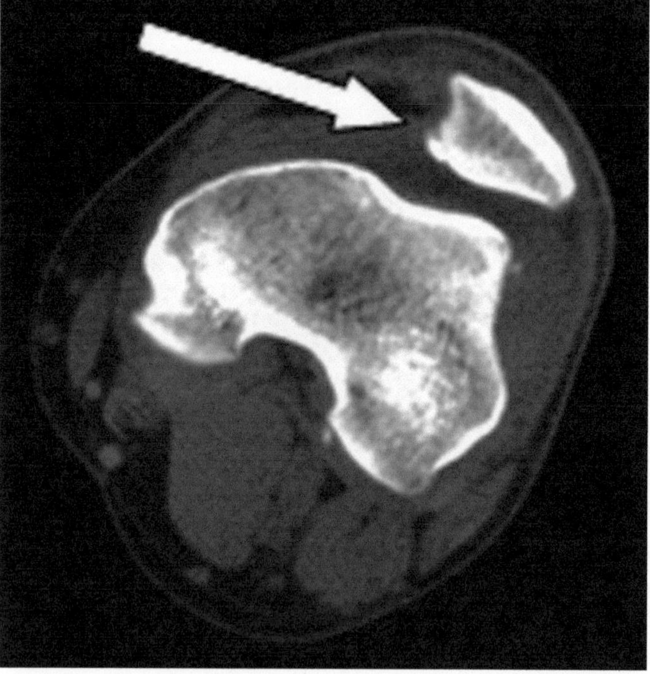

Fig. 10.14 CT through the patella shows a small avulsion of the patellar apex (*arrow*)

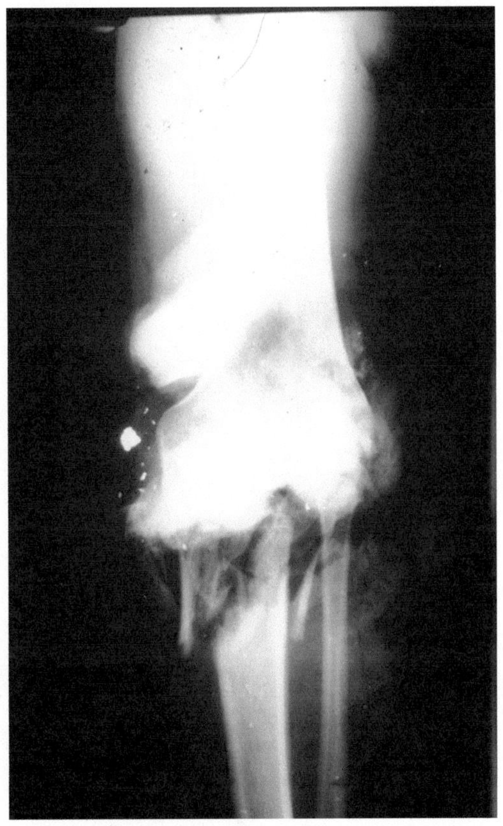

Fig. 10.15 This AP knee demonstrates tibial disruption from an RPG (Rocket Powered Grenade) to the knee. In addition to the comminuted fractures of the proximal tibia and fibula, the tibial plateau is essentially gone

X-ray of the knee was obtained to determine source of the fragment and demonstrated that the previously described popliteal fossa fragment was absent (see Figs. 10.18–10.22).

The Vietnam Vascular Registry showed that only 22 patients with known vascular trauma had missile emboli and of those, only four were to the pulmonary artery [4].

The next case has been well described by Riojas and Folio [5] and is that of a 42-year-old active duty male who jumped to exit his truck wearing body armor and weapons and felt a pop in his left knee with extreme pain. The patient then tried hopping on the other leg to get medical attention and felt a similar pop in the opposite leg with pain. He then proceeded to crawl to seek help. Eventually, he was picked up and taken to a combat hospital where plain radiographs were taken of both knees. See Figs. 10.23 and 10.24 for an example of patella alta, a high riding patella, bilaterally. A joint effusion was also noted. On MRI, disrupted patellar tendons were noted bilaterally (Figs. 10.2, 10.4 and 10.25).

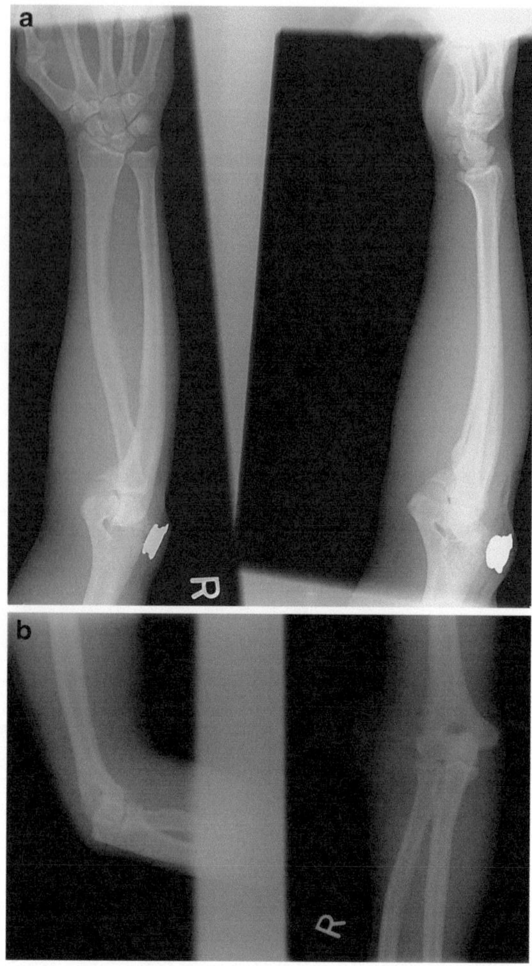

Fig. 10.16 (**a**) This airman reported to our emergency department with an open elbow wound from a 50 caliber fragment from a backfiring. Note the large fragment associated with subcutaneous emphysema. (**b**) The postoperative X-rays demonstrating the removed fragment, with some bone fragments remaining from impact to the bone

The last case represents an example of a common occurrence in the deployed military setting, however, to an extreme. This case has been well described by McKim and Folio [6] and represents a stress fracture in a soldier with continued unexplained pain (until imaging was obtained). This patient was a 28-year-old active duty U.S. Army combat soldier with progressive pain over his lower right leg that radiated to his knee joint for approximately 3 months with no history of direct trauma. Nonsteroidal anti-inflammatory medications provided temporary

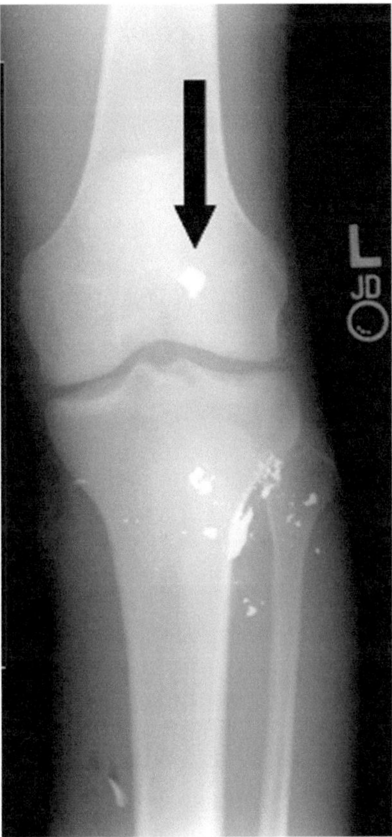

Fig. 10.17 AP knee showing multiple metallic fragments from the GSW of the navigator while in the helicopter. Note the fragment in the popliteal fossa (*arrow*). Case images are reprinted with permission from Military Medicine: International Journal of AMSUS

relief but did not improve his ambulatory pain. Plain X-rays were obtained and seen in Figs. 10.26–10.29.

The following case shows how 3D reformatting can help convey the seriousness of a ballistic injury to bone, especially when it is a weight bearing structure that can be difficult to repair, even in young, health soldiers. This troop was shot from below into his left lesser and greater trochanters on the left. Repair of this disruption can be difficult when evaluating the amount of destruction (Figs. 10.30–10.32).

Many blast injuries occurred to extremities because of exposure. This next example is representative of the destructive nature of explosions demonstrating disruption of the thumb and distal ulna, with several retained fragments. These types of injuries lead to significant destruction and often permanent disability and resultant deformity (Figs. 10.33 and 10.34).

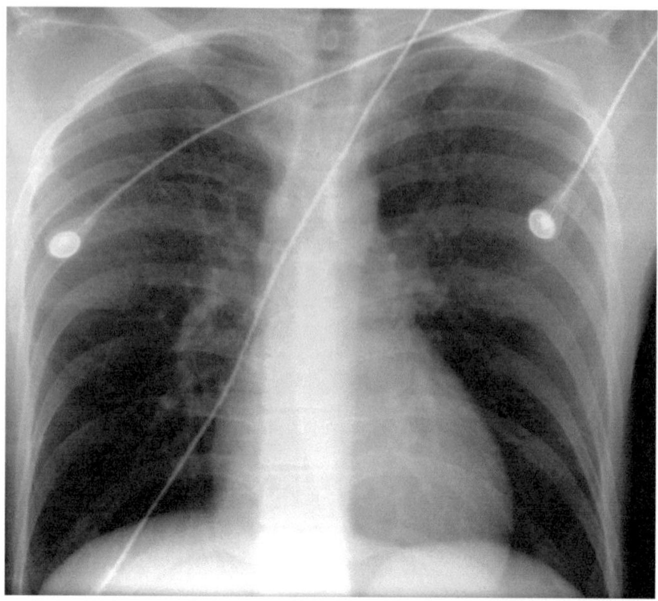

Fig. 10.18 Lateral knee also obtained before migration of the popliteal fragment

Fig. 10.19 Normal CXR obtained within minutes of the injury. No metallic fragments noted

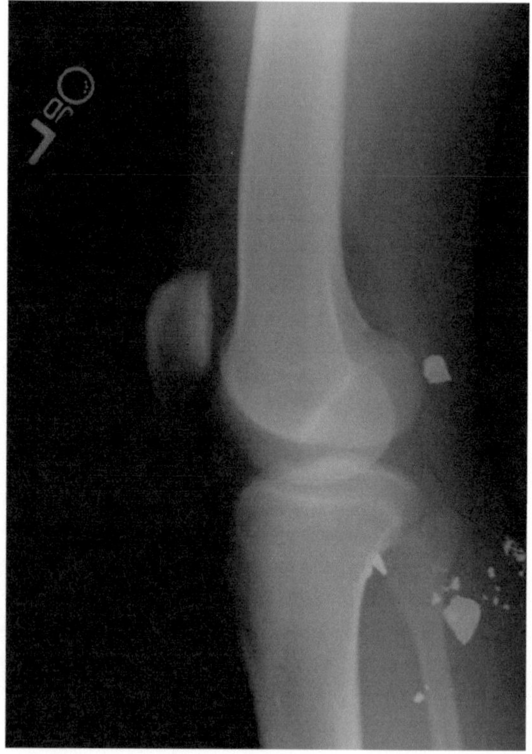

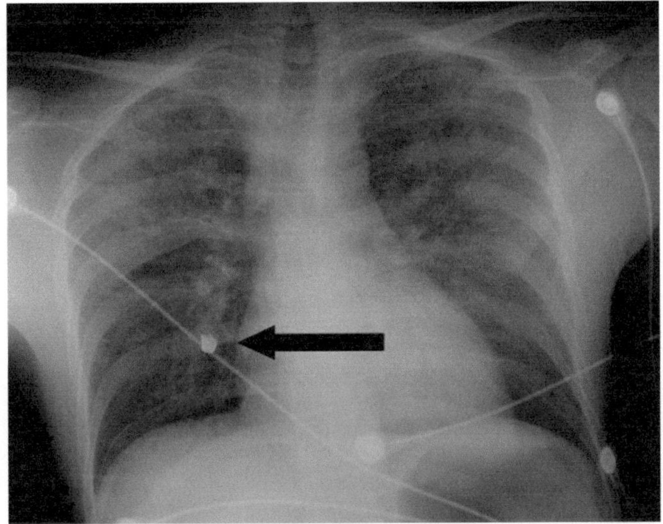

Fig. 10.20 Follow up CXR obtained when patient became hypoxic demonstrating fragment in right lower lung field

Fig. 10.21 Follow-up AP knee demonstrates absence of the previously seen fragment, supporting the migration of the projectile that embolized to the pulmonary artery

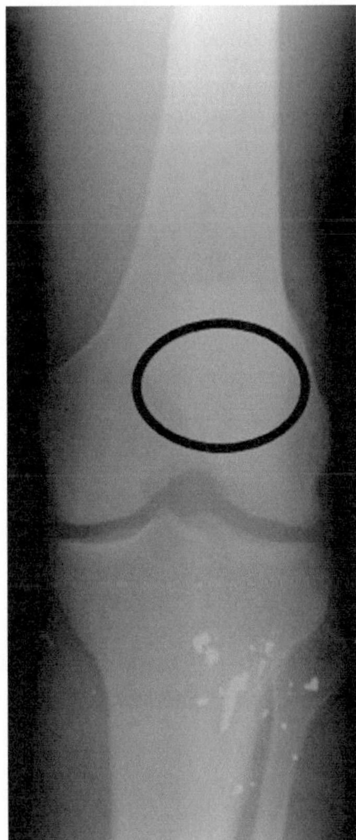

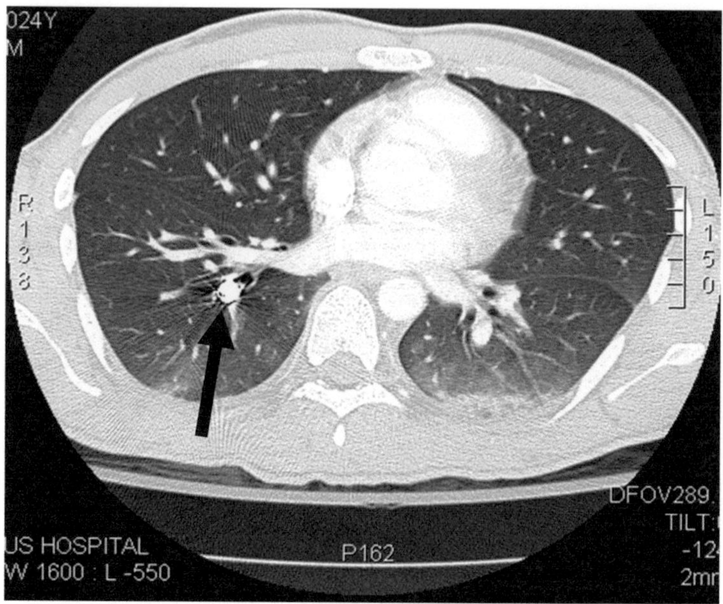

Fig. 10.22 CT with contrast verifying fragment migration to the right lower lobe pulmonary artery

Fig. 10.23 AP knee showing a high-riding patella, however, see the lateral that better demonstrates patella alta. Case images are reprinted with permission from Military Medicine: International Journal of AMSUS

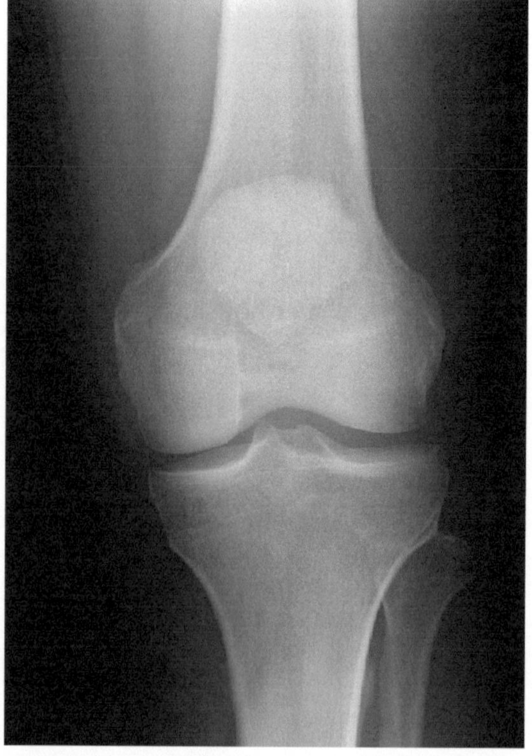

Fig. 10.24 Lateral knee
demonstrating patella alta

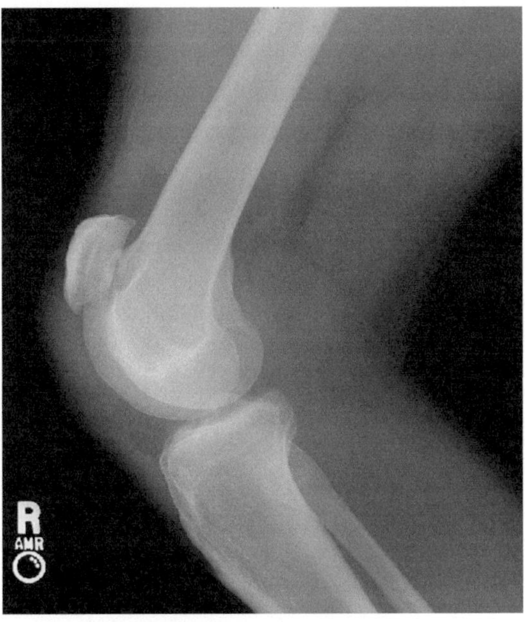

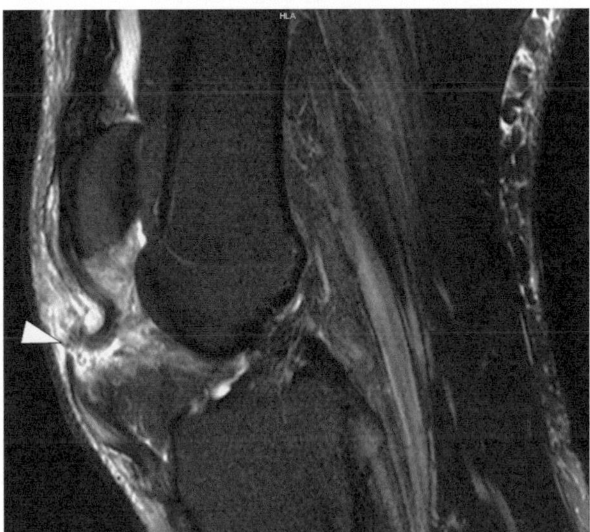

Fig. 10.25 T2-weighted sagittal MRI of the right knee. The patella tendon is retracted and
disrupted with associated increased signal representing inflammation around the tendon with
surrounding fluid

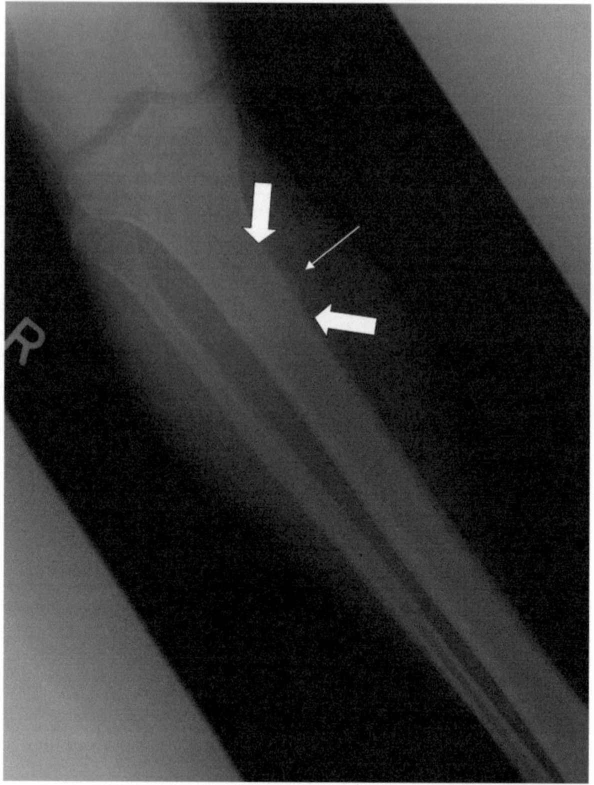

Fig. 10.26 Plain radiographs showing a classic appearance of a stress fracture of the tibia note the absence of any defined fracture lucency. Case images are reprinted with permission from Military Medicine: International Journal of AMSUS

Injuries are common occurrences even on the battlefield. This case highlights why workers dealing with heavy machinery should not wear rings in the workplace. This ring avulsion came from an aircraft maintenance airman that had his wedding ring caught in a cog that nearly amputated his finger off at that point (Figs. 10.35 and 10.36).

This next case again highlights a common occupational injury, from a nail gun while constructing a temporary structure for the new hospital. The nail gun accidently went off when it swung down and contacted his left knee. We did not obtain a single AP with the entire nail on it due to other war casualties in need of imaging. However, the surgeons had enough information to operate. The nail was firmly in place clinically, leading to the suspicion of bone impaction that was confirmed in surgery (Figs. 10.37–10.40).

One case not shown here, however, previously published, includes a new imaging processing technology that allows morphing of images over time to document

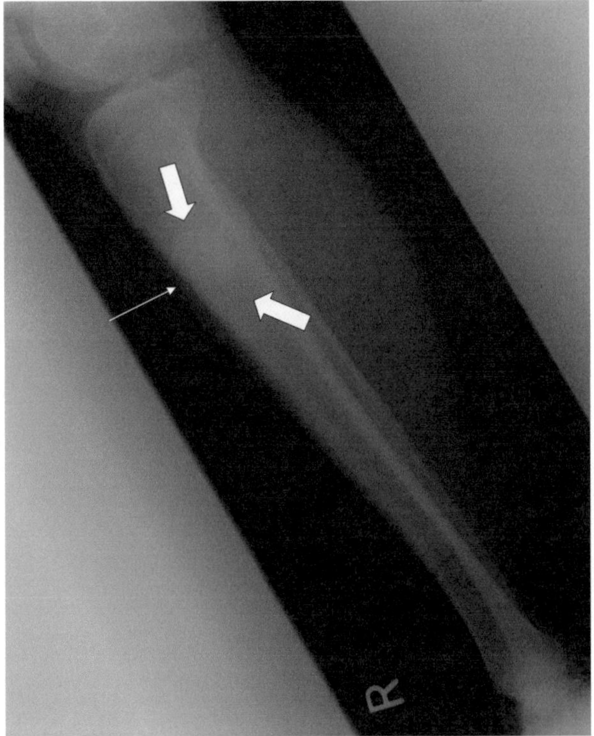

Fig. 10.27 Lateral demonstrates a periosteal reaction (*thin arrow*) along with a wide zone of transition band of increased density (*wide arrows*) commonly seen in tibial stress fractures

healing. Penska et al. demonstrate how a severe ballistic injury to the humerus shows miraculous repair over time [7]. Videos are available online for viewing of the healing of a severe humerus fracture from a GSW, and the rapid destruction of necrotizing fasciitis in another patient that was bitten by a Brown Recluse spider. This simple technology demonstrates to medical professionals and patients the effectiveness of external fixators and current treatment techniques.

10.2 Summary

This chapter should shed light on how imaging helps orthopedic surgeons manage skeletal trauma in combat. The radiologist can also guide surgeons and ED staff on priorities of imaging and optimal studies to be obtained depending on injury. Arterial injuries and limb salvageability are covered in another chapter. Although external fixation was not covered in detail here, this technology and its applications have helped save numerous extremities in recent years.

Fig. 10.28 CT coronal reformation of the stress fracture demonstrating the stress fracture with the periosteal reaction

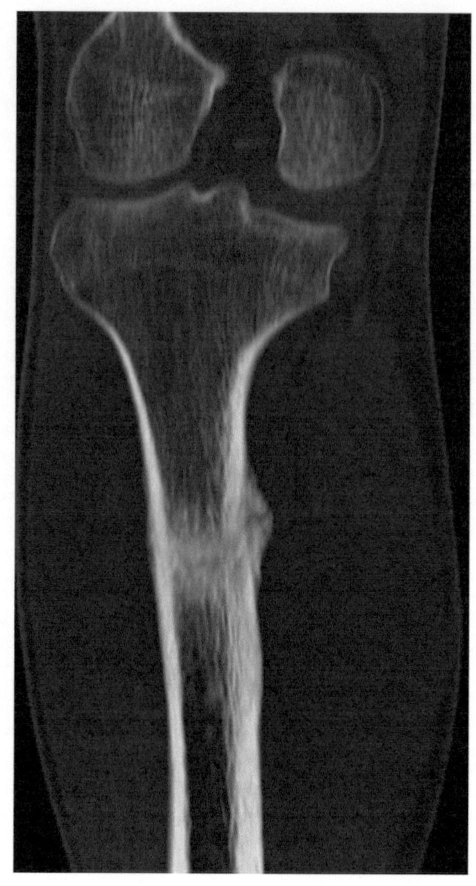

Fig. 10.29 Sagittal reformation CT of the stress fracture demonstrating a lucency running from anterior to posterior in the center of the stress fracture

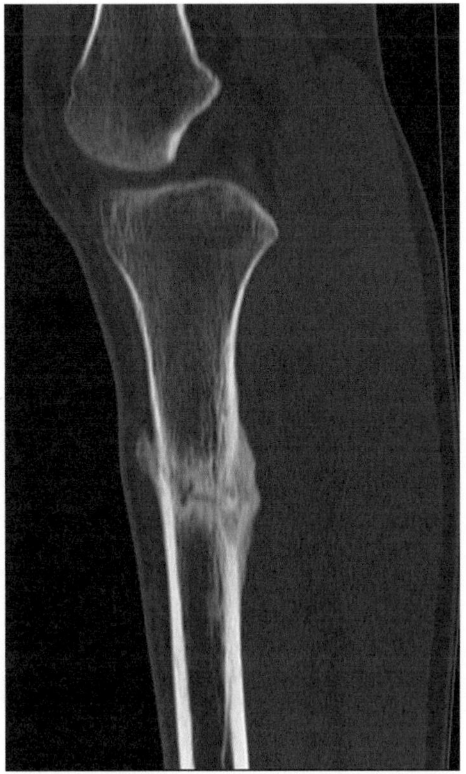

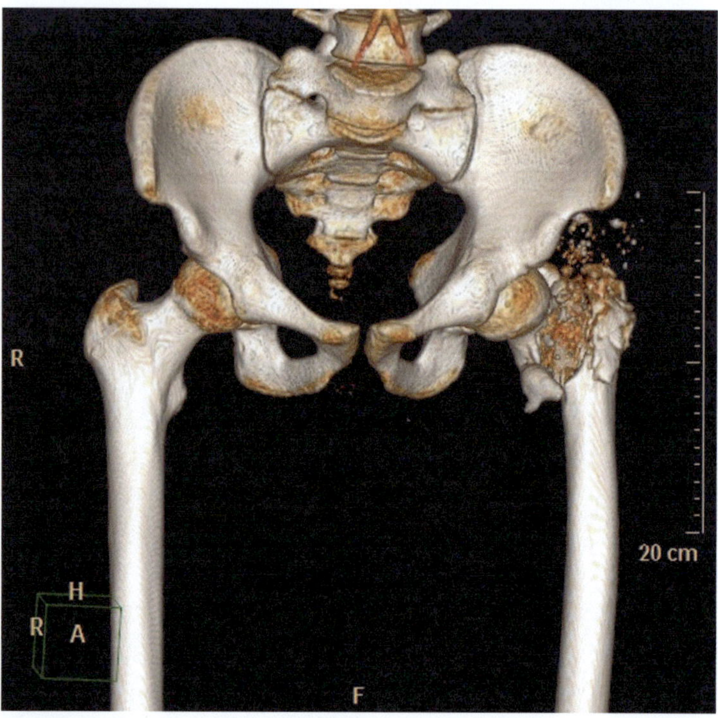

Fig. 10.30 This 3D CT shows the focal destructive effect on bone from a direct GSW from inferior to superior. Both the lesser and greater trochanters are disrupted into many pieces

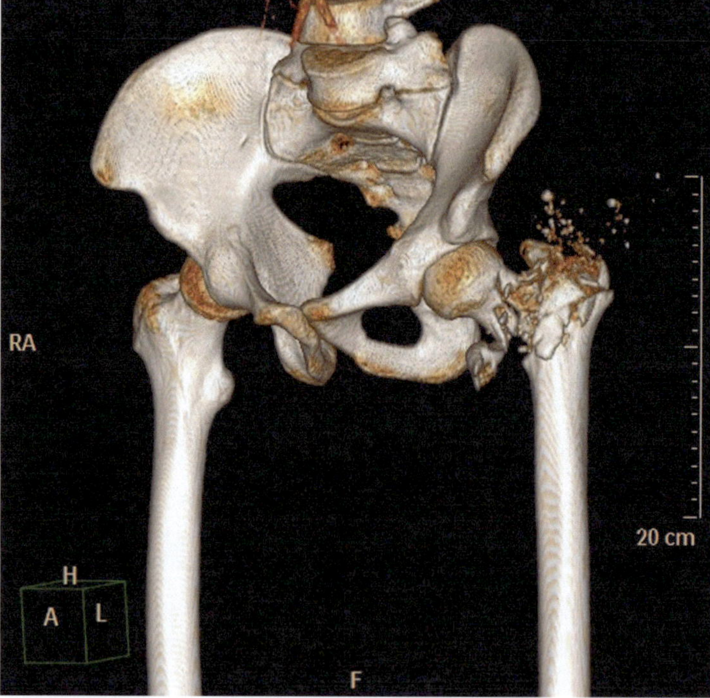

Fig. 10.31 Rotated 3D CT showing the destruction from another perspective

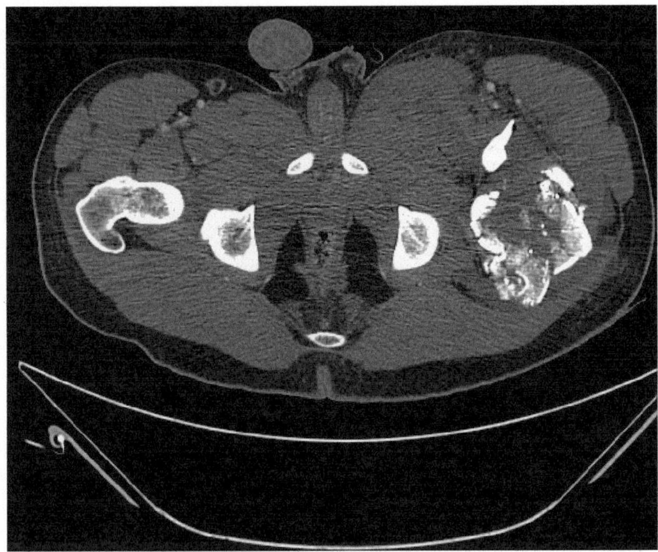

Fig. 10.32 Axial CT of damaged left trochanters also demonstrating soft tissue destruction, hematoma, however, major vascular integrity. The leg was salvaged, however, repair likely took some time with significant disability

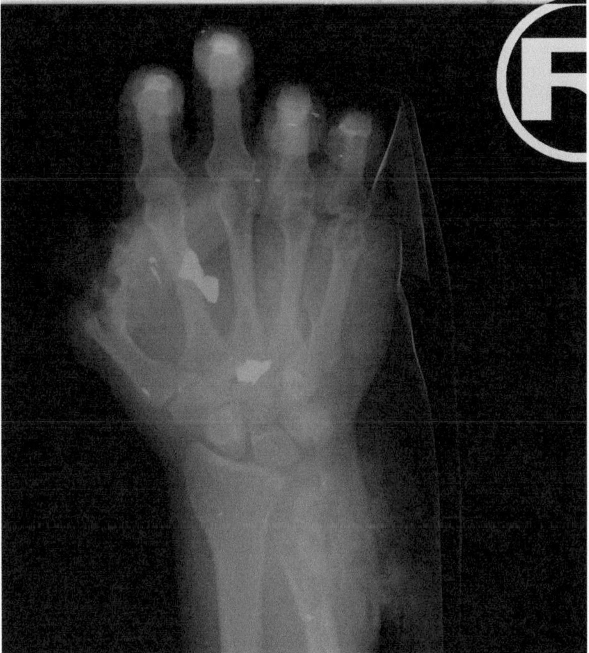

Fig. 10.33 AP right hand of a soldier in close proximity to a blast suffering near total amputation of his thumb. The thumb was amputated with a stump for some opposition possibilities

Fig. 10.34 Lateral demonstrating the fragment locations, one superficial posteriorly, the other within the carpals making removal more of a challenge. The ulna was able to be repaired to some degree

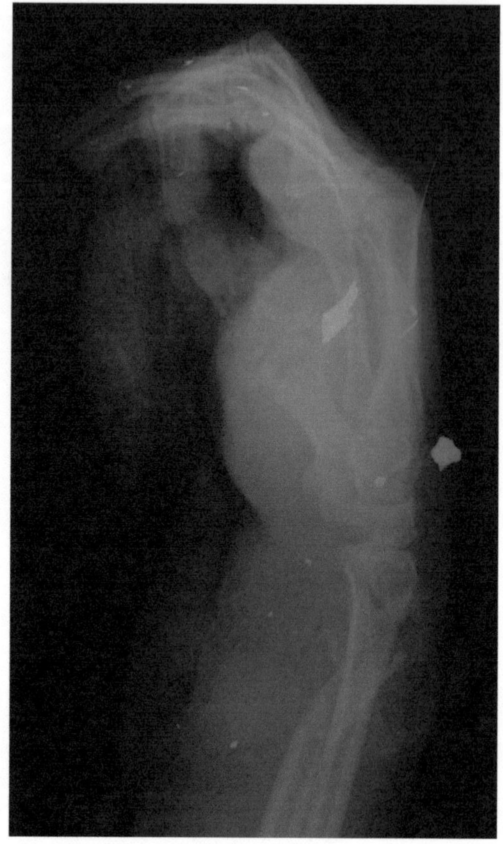

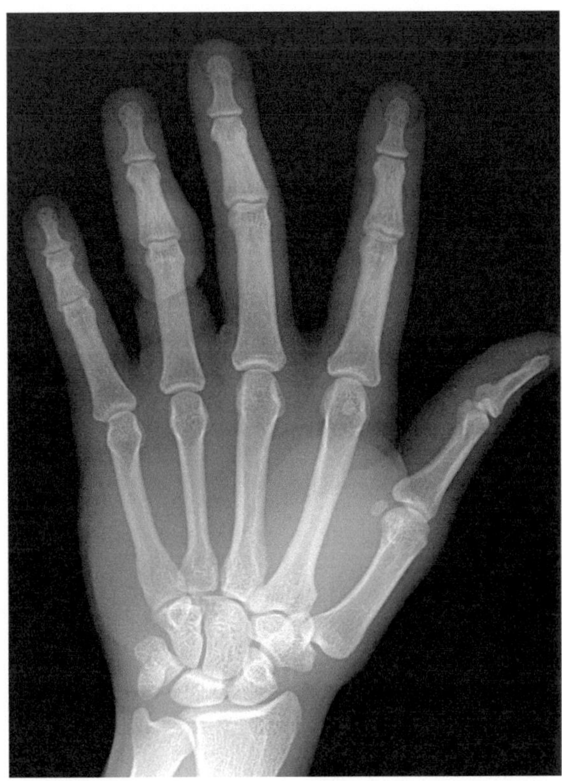

Fig. 10.35 Note the soft tissue defect in the shape of a ring on the ring finger

Fig. 10.36 The fourth digit was salvaged in this lucky aircraft maintainer, however, he could have easily lost his finger in the heavy machinery

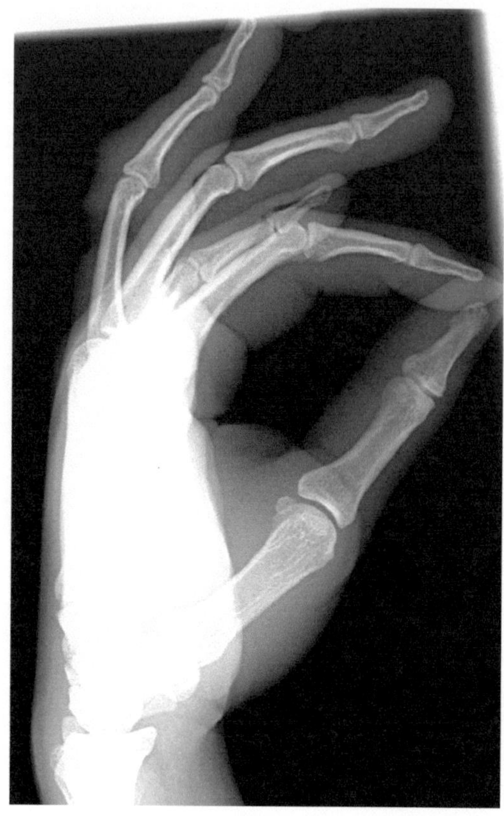

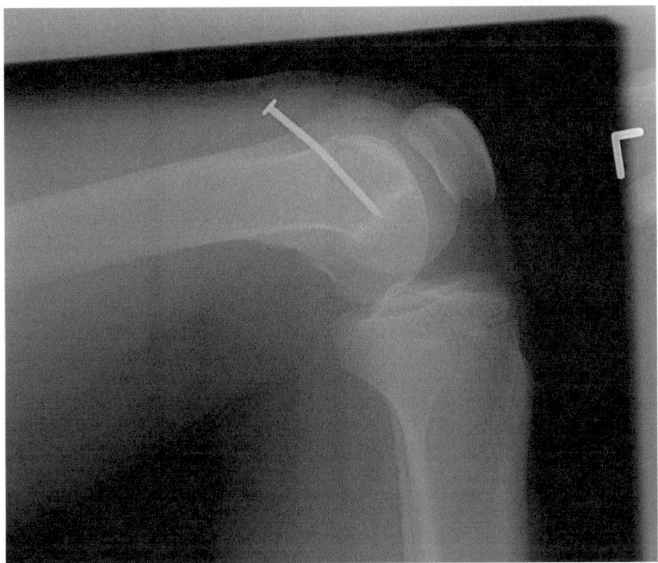

Fig. 10.37 Portable lateral knee showing nail overlying the distal femur

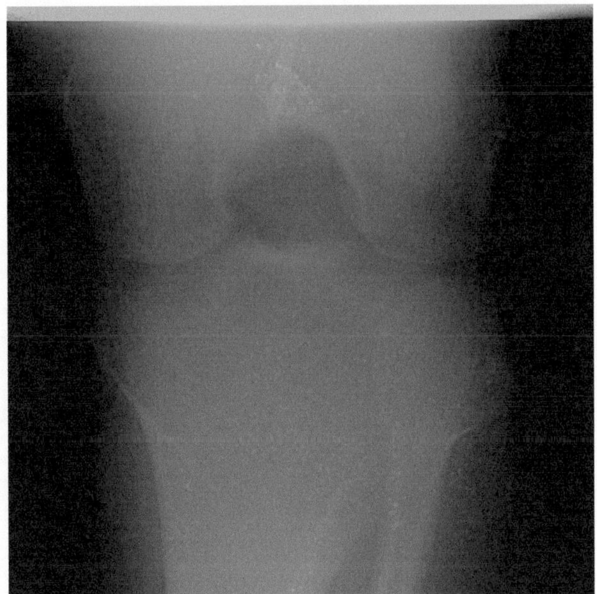

Fig. 10.38 Limited AP demonstrating nail tip nearing the intercondylar notch

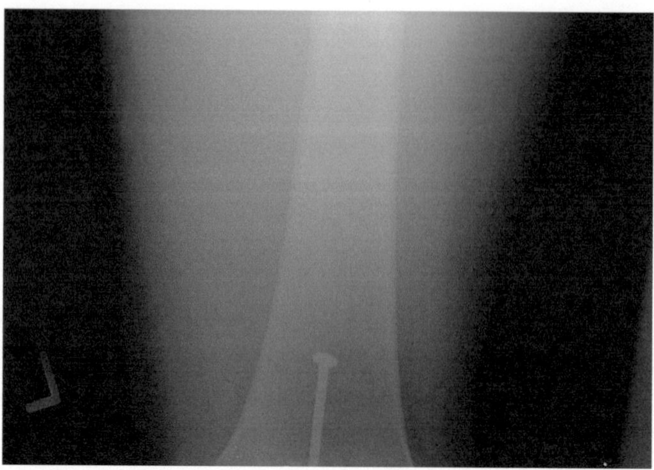

Fig. 10.39 Another AP centered higher verifying nail location in bone. Another AP to include whole nail was not able to be obtained in time due to other injuries of more serious nature

Fig. 10.40 Lateral knee postoperatively showing removal of nail without residual metal. Also note the subcutaneous emphysema in the soft tissues and joint space

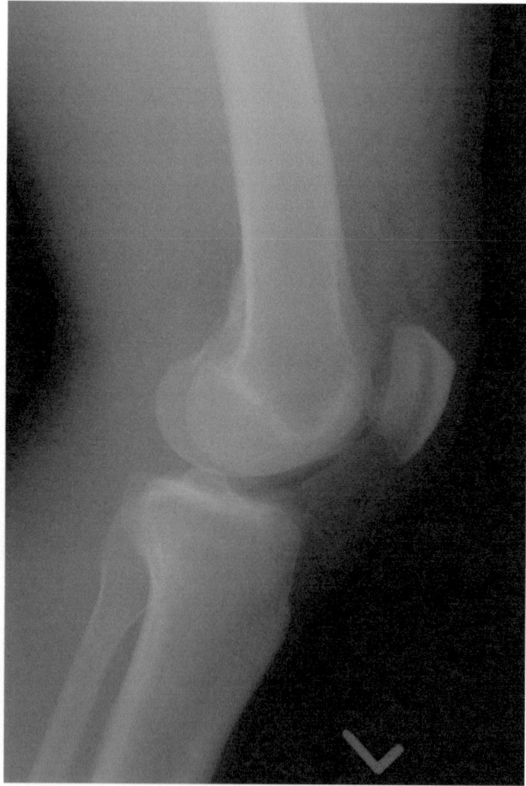

References

1. Lin DL, Kirk KL, Murphy KP, McHale KA, Doukas WC. Evaluation of orthopaedic injuries in Operation Enduring Freedom. J Orthop Trauma. 2004 Sep, 18(8 Suppl):S48–53.
2. Geiger S, McCormick F, Chou R, Wandel AG. War wounds: lessons learned from Operation Iraqi Freedom. Plast Reconstr Surg. 2008 Jul, 122(1):146–53.
3. Andrews C, Andrews K, Folio L. Venous fragment embolism to the pulmonary artery: a rare occurrence – case report and literature review of venous fragment embolization to the pulmonary artery. Mil Med. 2009 Sep, 174(9): iv–v.
4. Rich NM, Collins GJ Jr, Anderson CA et al. Missile emboli. J Trauma. 1978 Apr, 18(4):236–9.
5. Riojas R, Folio L. Bilateral patella tendon rupture in soldier in Iraq. Mil Med. 2009 Jul, 174(7): iii–iv.
6. McKim D, Folio L. Tibial stress fracture. Mil Med. 2008 Jun, 173(6):x–xi.
7. Penska K, Folio L, Bunger R. Medical applications of digital image morphing. J Digit Imaging. 2007 Feb 2. http://www.springerlink.com/content/0574n3u78tt84vku/fulltext.pdf or http://dx.doi.org/10.1007/s10278-006-1050-5 (both accessed Dec 09).